A PRELIMINARY DESIGN FOR A UNIVERSAL PATIENT MEDICAL RECORD

A PRELIMINARY DESIGN FOR A UNIVERSAL PATIENT MEDICAL RECORD

RE-ENGINEERING HEALTH CARE

MICHAEL R. MCGUIRE

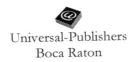

Universal-Publishers
Boca Raton

A Preliminary Design for a Universal Patient Medical Record:
Re-engineering Health Care

Universal-Publishers
Boca Raton, Florida • USA
2010
ISBN-10: 1-59942-872-5
ISBN-13: 978-1-59942-872-7

www.universal-publishers.com

Library of Congress Cataloging-in-Publication Data
McGuire, Michael R., 1945-
A preliminary design for a universal patient medical record
: re-engineering health care / Michael R. McGuire.
    p. ; cm.
Includes bibliographical references.
ISBN-13: 978-1-59942-872-7 (pbk. : alk. paper)
ISBN-10: 1-59942-872-5 (pbk. : alk. paper)
 1. Medical records--Standards. I. Title.
[DNLM: 1. Medical Record Linkage. 2. Delivery of
Health Care--trends. 3. Medical Records Systems,
Computerized. WX 173 M4776p 2010]
 R864.M37 2010
 610.285--dc22

                                    2009052100

ACKNOWLEDGEMENTS

Firstly, I would like to thank my many past colleagues at Kaiser Permanente in Northern California, an HMO, from whom I learned a lot about health care, health care computing, and life. These colleagues include David Rentz, Gloria Lawrence, Connie Compton Balsley, Don Bloomstine, Dr. Ted Cooper, Dr. Richard Fury, Joe Loverti, Louise Yuen, Becky Denevan, Kuruvilla Mathen, and many others.

I would also like to thank the many fine universities in the San Francisco Bay Area that provide extension courses in medicine, biology and computing for interested students such as me: the University of California Santa Cruz Extension for its many computer science courses; UC San Francisco for its Mini Medical School; and the UC Berkeley Extension for its biology, psychology, and medicine-related courses. I would also like to thank the Learning Company for its Great Courses video series in anatomy, psychology and medicine.

Most significantly, I would like to thank my wife Bonnie for her encouragement in pursuing my hobby of a universal patient medical record. And I would like to thank God for Bonnie and me getting older and sicker, and thus learning what it means to be patients.

Please note that I am not a physician and thus any medical examples in this book clearly are not meant to be used to treat or diagnose any medical condition. Examples come from medical conditions I have personally experienced or from referenced studies as noted.

CONTENTS

I

INTRODUCTION

This book proposes development of a universal patient medical record (UPR) that provides a complete medical history for the patient and that enables access to all the patient's medical records no matter where they are located.

It is assumed that in the future most all health care organizations will use electronic patient record systems (EPRs) that automate their patient medical records. An electronic medical record system will allow clinicians to enter clinical information while seeing patients and may send orders and receive back results and other information from automated ancillary systems (e.g., test results from clinical laboratory systems, admissions from hospital admission systems, etc). Patients' medical records for a health care organization with an EPR will thus be stored in the health care organization's EPR. The universal patient medical record for a patient would be created by combining information from EPR systems from all the health care organizations where the patient was seen for care.

Why develop such a universal patient medical record that would be available to all clinicians caring for a patient no matter where the clinician is located? One should be developed because it would benefit patients, benefit payers and benefit mankind, and because it is inevitable.

Health care today is largely oriented toward short-term treatment of a medical condition and upon a typical patient with that medical condition. I predict this will change in the near future: medical care will become more long-term oriented. Care will be more personalized to the individual patient. Besides treating disease, medical care will prevent disease and promote wellness and a healthy longevity without disease. These changes in care will result in a need for an always-available, complete medical, prevention and wellness history for a patient that is accurate and up-to-date, available to any clinician caring for the patient, no matter where the patient is being seen for care.

A patient's medical, prevention and wellness history would include *biomarkers* for disease or health, where biomarkers have been defined by the National Institutes of Health as "cellular, biochemical, molecular, or genetic characteristics or alterations by which a normal, abnormal, or simply biologic process can be recognized, or monitored" (NIH 2000). An individual's genome could provide permanent biomarkers while other biomarkers may change over time. Through biomarkers, diseases and wellness could be predicted. A universal patient medical record is a place where such biomarkers for an individual could be stored. Biomarkers identify the inner workings of an individual's cells and thus enable diagnoses, preventions and treatments to be tailored to the individual.

When medical records were first used, the medical records were on paper and medical care was most often performed by a physician who worked individually in the care of a patient. With managed care, national health care, and the greater mobility of people moving from place to place, care is no longer given by an individual physician but by many. Even when care occurs in a single health care organization, care is often given by multiple physicians, with a primary care physician referring the patient to a specialist physician for any complex medical condition, and care is often given by teams of clinicians, both physicians and non-physicians. There is a need for a universal patient medical record that supports communication between these many clinicians, whether the clinicians work together or independently in providing a patient's care or work in different health care organizations. A universal patient medical record should thus be centered around an individual, not a health care organization nor any single clinician.

Through a universal patient medical record, visits involving the same medical condition could be combined into a "case", both supporting team-based care and continuity-of-care whether care is provided by a team or an individual physician over a significant period of time. Documentation of care plans based upon standards of care for the medical condition and documentation of the results of care (outcomes) could be included within the case documentation, enabling standards of care to be evaluated based upon comparative effectiveness.

Today, each physician is restricted to providing care in a very specific geographic location of the world. With telecommunications and telemedicine, this need not be so. Health care could be accomplished by a physician located anywhere in the world and a patient located anywhere else in the world. Thus, there is a need for remotely located caregivers to be able to concurrently access the same patient medical record in the care of a patient.

As evidenced by the HIV/AIDS and influenza pandemics and by global warming, the health of each person in the world can be affected by what happens in other parts of the world. There are too few physicians in the world, too few nurses, and too few other health care workers. The world must make better use of all its health care workers. This can be facilitated by a universal patient medical record.

There would be a complete, immediately available, medical record. When a patient showed up for care with identification in an emergency department, even when unconscious, a universal patient medical record could provide the health history for the patient, informing clinicians of drug allergies, significant health problems, current medications or other information that could improve care or potentially save the patient's life.

The universal patient medical record together with the EPR systems could save money in many ways, including identifying when billing was inconsistent with the care given. Discharge activities could be done concurrently, quicker and thus with less cost. Public health organizations, insurance companies, the patient's primary care physician, or other interested parties with a need-to-know could be sent information on patient care after care is given or while care is being given, providing information quicker, potentially reducing fraud, providing better care, and quickly identifying public health problems before they get worse. Costs for paper, diagnostic image film, and associated labor, time, and space to transport and store them can be saved as well as saving costs due to medical errors caused by misplacement, unavailability or unreadability of such non-automated documents. The universal patient medical record could support clinical trials of standards of care to identify standards of care that produce the best outcomes for the least cost. Through the universal patient medical record, diagnostic tests and prescriptions which are duplicated or inconsistent with care could be identified—in particular, identification of duplicate prescriptions could be used to identify narcotics abuse by patients.

With automation, the universal patient medical record could use sophisticated approaches to security and privacy.

For example, researchers might be able to only get medical information that does not reveal the identity of the patient (an approach consistent with HIPAA). Patients might be able to exclude some categories of mental health, wellness or other information from the universal patient medical record for view by others.

The universal patient medical record could also be designed for the patient, enabling the patient to comply with physician advice and orders, and enabling the patient to verify that advice given by the physician was indeed given, that the encounter did indeed occur, and that services stated indeed were provided.

To summarize, with a universal patient medical record:

- Better patient care could be provided that avoids medical mistakes due to lack of information resulting from the unavailability of a patient's medical record.

- There would be a single, complete automated patient medical record, rather than many fragmented ones.

- Communications between all types of clinicians would be enhanced, whether they worked on a single treatment for a patient, over many treatments, or over the patient's lifetime.

- Continuity-of-care and team-based care would be supported by use of cases that combine visits for the same medical condition. Cases could include overall care plans and the outcomes of care, making it easier for the evaluation of care plans based upon standards of care, and identifying best practices based upon comparative effectiveness. Biomarkers related to the medical condition that could identify the best treatment for the medical condition could be stored with the case (e.g., the genetics of the patient's breast cancer).

- There would a single place to permanently store the lifestyles, environmental conditions, and disease and wellness biomarkers for an individual. There could then be greater emphasis on individualized care and preventive care, and diseases could be prevented before they occur.

- The lifestyles, environmental conditions, and biomarkers that predict diseases and wellness could be better determined as a result of a research database derived from these complete medical records.

- Health care workers could work across borders and provide consultation and mentoring even when the health care workers were located remotely from each other, or remotely from the patient.

- Public health agencies, clinicians and the public could be more quickly informed about public health problems.

- The patient could better comply with physician directives and verify that medical record information was correct.

- Privacy and security of patient information could be protected while providing adequate information for care, public health, payments and medical research.

- Money could be saved.

This book is titled *A Preliminary Design for a Universal Patient Medical Record*. A preliminary design is a first draft of how to construct a software and hardware system. A preliminary design's principal uses are to verify that requirements for the system as determined by the users of the system have been satisfied, and to serve as a framework and initial specifications for the final design.

Since no requirements for the universal patient medical record have yet been determined by its users (physicians, public health workers, researchers, the government, software/hardware designers, etc.), I have assumed an initial set of requirements of the system and have based my preliminary design on these requirements. This preliminary design of a universal patient medical record could serve as a starting point for gathering of the actual user requirements for such a system and creating an actual preliminary, and then final, design for such a system.

Since a universal patient medical record must be built for health care tomorrow as well as today, chapter 2 of this book predicts how health care will change in the future.

Chapter 3 identifies a set of requirements for a universal patient medical record that would result in improvement of health care both today and tomorrow and presents a preliminary design of a universal patient medical record based upon these requirements.

The basis for my requirements for a universal patient medical record are that health care in the future will provide the greatest health benefits for patients while being much more efficient and cost-effective than it is today, i.e., creating the greatest value for the patient health care dollar. In the *New England Journal of Medicine*, Dr. Michael Porter presented his ideas for health care reform based upon the same goal of creating the greatest value for the patient. Chapter 4 summarizes Dr. Porter's ideas for health care reform and identifies how health care would have to be re-engineered to use a universal patient medical record to implement these reforms.

Throughout this book, words in italics are defined in the glossary.

2

HEALTH CARE TODAY AND TOMORROW

2.1 Health Care Today

Since a universal patient medical record would be enduring, it should be built both for health care today and tomorrow.

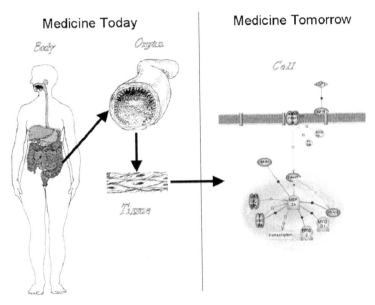

Figure 1 Medicine today and medicine tomorrow.

Medical care today—see figure 1—involves a clinician interviewing the patient; the clinician, anatomic pathology and the clinical laboratory looking at organs and tissues of the body of the patient to identify pathological conditions;

the clinician diagnosing and treating the medical condition; the clinician giving the patient advice on how the patient can maintain or improve his or her health; and the clinician prescribing medications, or performing or ordering other interventions.

Medical care tomorrow will function as it does today, but it will also look deeper into the chemistry within individual cells and signaling between cells to identify individual differences between patients with a particular medical condition. Care will thus be more personalized to the patient resulting in more effective treatments.

2.2 Health Care Tomorrow

I predict that health care will change in the following ways in the future:

- **Molecular medicine:** When clinicians look at the body at the cellular level, not just the tissue level, they may be able to diagnosis diseases with greater specificity (e.g., the diagnosis might be HER2-positive breast cancer instead of just breast cancer), and they may be able to determine the likelihood of a disease occurring in a currently healthy patient.

- **Team-based care and greater continuity-of-care:** In the future, there will be greater use of team care, which will result in saving money and providing greater continuity-of-care for a patient.

- **Preventive care:** In the future there will be greater use of preventive care with biomarkers being used to identify when preventive care is most beneficial and cost effective.

- **Wellness:** Lifestyles will be correlated with rates of disease. Education, together with a greater scientific understanding of the brain and how humans make decisions, will be used to change lifestyles.

- **Patient values and non-compliance:** Because of a patient's life situation or a patient's attitude or because of the complexity of proper use of medications, proper care may be provided by a clinician but the patient may not comply with the clinician's dictates. In the future, there will be greater use of non-clinicians to overcome these compliance impediments, including pharmacists, counselors, psychologists and patient educators. Also there will be greater use of written communication with the patient to enhance compliance.

- **Multiple medical conditions:** There will be better care for multiple medical conditions, including when care crosses multiple medical specialties.

- **Other Changes**

2.2.1 Molecular Medicine

See figure 1. Medicine today is performed at the organ and tissue level with diseases, treatments and preventive medicine working primarily with organs and tissues. Medicine tomorrow will also be at the cellular level, with differences in the functioning of the cells within a tissue identifying a disease, healthy or possible pre-disease condition. (*Systems biology* is study of biological systems at the cellular level.)

Cells function by chemical reactions that occur within the cells and by communication between cells. Figure 2 shows an example of the chemical reactions within a cell, showing what occurs in a muscle or fat cell as a result of the cell encountering insulin.

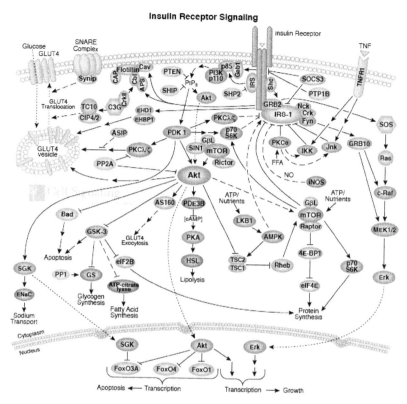

Figure 2 Example of cell signaling and interactions within a cell. (Pathway diagram reproduced courtesy of Cell Signaling Technology, Inc. (www.cellsignal.com)).

A cell has receptors embedded in its cell wall (membrane) or in the cytoplasm of a cell (the interior) that bind hormone, neurotransmitter or drug molecules. In this example, the molecule is a hormone, an insulin molecule. As a result of this binding of an insulin molecule with an insulin receptor, chemical reactions occur within the cell. For example, for muscle or fat cells, insulin causes an influx of glucose into the cell. These chemical reactions may involve the cell nucleus that contains the genome.

A cell, the smallest structure capable of basic life processes, is simply a complex chemical factory. The cell has receptors on its outside. Hormone molecules (such as insulin) or drug molecules can bind with the cell's receptors which initiate chemical reactions within the cell. The nucleus within a cell contains DNA (the genome) which forms a template for creating polypeptides that can fold and combine with other molecules or polypeptides to form proteins; proteins are involved in reactions and transport activities within the cell. Some proteins may be created automatically by the cell on an on-going basis, while some may be created only when chemical reactions occur within the cell as a result of a hormone, neurotransmitter or drug molecule binding to a receptor. Chemical reactions within a cell could result in the cell secreting a hormone that provides a signal to another cell (e.g., the insulin molecule in figure 2 that binds with the receptor of the muscle or fat cell came from a pancreas cell).

A *hormone*, a chemical created by one of your body's cells, is a way that cells within your body communicate with each other, with the hormone matching a receptor on a different cell, for example causing a chemical reaction in the receiving cell.

Neurotransmitters are chemicals that enable communication between neurons. Chemicals called neurotransmitters are released by a neuron to communicate with other neurons that have receptors very close to the release of the neurotransmitter; the small distance between the releasing neuron and receptor neuron is called a *synapse*.

Drugs are created to bind with receptors or affect neurotransmitters. In this way, drugs can change what happens within cells of the human body.

Figure 3 is a cartoon diagram of cell receptors. A receptor is most often itself a protein—a protein embedded in the cell membrane of the cell. Cells of different types (e.g., liver cell, pancreas cell, etc.) could have receptors which are totally different from each other, could have some receptors that are the same, or could have similar receptors that are different but are able to bind the same hormone or drug.

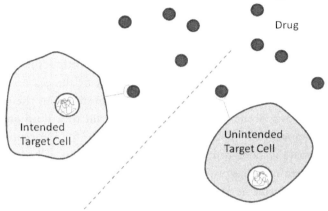

Figure 3 Cell receptors.

A cell that has a receptor that binds with a particular drug or hormone is called a "target cell" for that drug or hormone. As shown in figure 3, a drug that is meant to bind with a receptor of a particular type of cell—a intended target cell such as the prostate cell—may also bind with a receptor on another type of cell—an unintended target cell such as a liver cell. This is one reason drug side effects occur.

On the other hand, a particular drug might bind only to a receptor on the intended target cell (e.g., prostate cells) and not bind to receptors on other cells. This explains how a drug can be created that has an effect on a specific type of cell and not others (e.g., a drug to relax prostate muscle to enhance urinary flow).

Molecule-receptor interactions could be more complicated: For example, one type of molecule could bind with a receptor causing no internal cell chemical reaction but could result in blocking out these receptors from molecules that could cause chemical reactions. A molecule could also interact with a receptor, changing its configuration and thus changing the way the receptor works.

The study of the signaling between cells and the interworkings of cells for purposes of medical care is referred to as *molecular medicine*. *Genomics*, the study of the *genome*—the blueprint for creation of proteins within the interior of the cell—is part of molecular medicine; in particular, errors in the genome could result in cancer. *Personalized medicine* is diagnosing and treating patients based upon the interworkings of their cells resulting in diagnoses and treatments tailored for the individual patient.

Somatic cells are all the cells in the human body excluding reproductive cells (eggs and sperm). A general category of somatic cells in the human body are *adult stem cells* as opposed to non-stem cells. A *stem cell* is "a cell that can incur unlimited division and which has the potential to differentiate into other types of cells." For example, an adult stem cell might be able to produce other adult stem cells and non-stem cells upon division while a non-stem cell would either not be able to divide at all or would only be able to divide to produce other non-stem cells for a limited number of generations.

For a particular organ, there are often many non-stem cells and a smaller number of stem cells; for example, when part of a liver is removed, it grows back which appears to be due to the activation of liver stem cells (Sell 1990). Often the adult stem cells are hard to distinguish from the non-stem cells. Some authorities contend that cancer occurs in the adult stem cells, not the non-stem cells (Wade 2006).

A type of stem cell that occurs in an embryo is an *embryonic stem cell* (ESC) that has the potential to divide to produce **all** other types of human cells. Somatic stem cells occurring within the human body, adult stem cells, can only divide to produce a much limited number of types of other cells. Scientists have been able to reproduce ESC-like stem cells from adult skin stem cells and neurons; these new cells were termed induced pluripotent stem cells (iPSCs) (Kim et al. 2009).

Every cell in a particular human's body has the same genome and set of genes, with genes being sections of the genome that are templates for producing polypeptides that fold and combine to produce proteins. Embryonic stem cells *differentiate* into many different types of cells. This differentiation is done by particular genes being turned off for a particular type of cell (e.g.., differentiation of embryonic stem cells to produce a liver cell); in this case, turning off of genes occurs through *epigenetic processes*, i.e., by mechanisms other than changes in the underlying DNA sequence (Wikipedia 2009). Differentiation of cells in embryos results from signaling between cells with different signaling dependent upon the location of the cells in the embryo (Microsoft ® Encarta ® 2007).

The DNA in a cell is wrapped around spool-like protein structures called *histones*. *Epigenetic* changes in the DNA that turn off or turn on genes (i.e., keep them from being or allow them to be *transcribed* and thus to be *expressed* to produce proteins) involve at least two phenomena: (1) the physical blocking of genes by the packaging of the genome on histones, which may cause a gene to not be transcribed, and (2) the addition of methyl groups to some cytosine bases in the genome—termed *DNA methylation* (Watters 2006). These two phenomena are related: the methyl groups are what change the histone packaging and cause suppression of gene expression.

Besides being responsible for creation of the different types of cells in the human body from embryonic stem cells, epigenetic changes occur in all cells in the human body over their lifetime. Random changes in genes in the genome, *mutations*, together with epigenetic changes in cells could result in the occurrence of cancer. According to reference (Pelengaris and Khan 2006), "Cancers arise by the stepwise accumulation of mutations and epigenetic factors that alter gene expression to confer cancer properties on the cell. The presence of inherited cancer-causing mutations will give a would-be cancer cell a head start, but somatic mutations and epigenetic alterations are still needed for cancer development."

DNA (*deoxyribonucleic acid*) is a long double-stranded molecule in the genome of a cell. RNA (*ribonucleic acid*) is a shorter single-stranded molecule that is used to transcribe genes to produce polypeptides by combining various types of amino acids. RNAi (*RNA interference*) is a naturally occurring micro-RNA that can be used to *knock down* a protein, in other words to stop the protein from being expressed. RNAi is used by drug companies to determine what happens to cells if a particular protein that is normally expressed is not expressed and upon positive results could identify to the drug company to create a drug that could have the same effect; in the future RNAi could also potentially be used in drugs to fight diseases by stopping protein expression in a cell.

Living things that can cause disease, and also viruses, have either DNA or RNA. Some misfolded proteins (*prions*)—containing neither DNA or RNA—can also cause disease (bovine spongiform encephalopathy, Creutzfeldt-

Jakob disease, and scrapie); some researchers suspect that prion-like proteins may be also be involved in more major diseases such as Alzheimer's and Parkinson's diseases. (Miller 2009)

Today, drug companies are interested in the cellular level of medicine to identify drug targets, receptors on cells for their drugs that initiate chemical reactions of desired types within the desired type of cell. These receptors and chemical reactions may apply generally to many patients or just to a subset of patients. In the future, patient care tailored to a patient, personalized medicine, will be based upon these differences in cell receptors and inter-workings of cells.

The importance of molecular and personalized medicine is that (1) there could be a more precise diagnosis of a disease enabling determination of the best treatment for the disease, (2) a disease or pre-disease could potentially be identified at an earlier stage enabling the disease to be treated before the disease becomes severe or before it becomes untreatable, (3) there would be new treatments and medications tailored for a more precise diagnosis including medications based upon the individual's genetics, (4) in some cases it can be determined whether a particular drug can benefit or will have side effects for a patient (e.g., the CYP2D6 gene variant in individuals can determine whether codeine has no effect on pain in the individual or conversely, whether an otherwise normal dose of codeine could lead to morphine intoxication in the individual (Thorn, Klein and Altman 2009)), (5) preventive measures could be taken for a patient targeted toward that patient's predisposition for a disease, and (6) for some life-threatening or life-altering genetic diseases, *gene therapy* could potentially cure the disease. More precise diagnosis of a disease will either change disease coding or require the addition of new biomarkers to the current disease coding (e.g., this breast cancer is HER2 positive). *Pharmacogenetics* (Wikipedia 2009) is "the study of genetic variation that gives rise to differing responses to drugs." *Gene therapy* (Microsoft ® Encarta ® 2007) is "manipulating genes in cells—often using viruses—in order to produce proteins that change the functions of a cell."

Support for molecular medicine and personalized medicine should be provided in future patient medical records and any universal patient medical record.

2.2.2 Team-Based Care

David Lawrence MD, the former CEO of Kaiser Permanente, contends that a big change in medical care in the future will be greater use of teams to provide care. (Lawrence 2003)

Team care is not so important for acute care, even though there are indeed teams involved in acute care: a physician, a nurse taking vital signs, a person taking a blood sample, a clinical laboratory and a pharmacist. Team care is more important for chronic conditions and for any care over an extended period of time, e.g., care for a cancer.

A medical *intervention* is "an action that produces an effect or that is intended to alter the course of a disease process." An *outcome* is "a natural or artificially designed point in the care of an individual or population suitable for assessing the effect of an intervention, or lack of intervention, on the natural history of a condition" (McCallum 1993). Health care should strive for medical *interventions* that produce the best outcomes, called *evidence-based care.*

Team care would be haphazard unless it is organized. Team care could be organized by (1) a clinician creating a care plan for the medical condition at the beginning of care identifying expected interventions and follow-up visits together with *red flags* (changes in the medical condition to watch for) based upon the where the patient currently is in the life cycle of the medical condition, with the care plan modified as necessary, (2) planning for the most cost-effective caregivers as needed over the time of the care plan together with the use of equipment and medications that provides the greatest benefit for a patient without over-treatment (Mahar 2006), and (3) the clinician identifying intermediate or final outcomes of care. The care plan would be based upon a *standard-of-care* for the medical condition, where a *standard-of-care* is "a diagnostic and treatment process that a clinician should follow for a certain type of patient, illness, or clinical circumstance" (BSCS 2003). *Best practice* for a disease is "the standard-of-care that produces the best outcomes with the least harm with consideration of the cost-effectiveness of the care compared to other standards of care for the disease"; such a standard-of-care is sometimes called the "gold standard."

Well organized team-based care has the advantages that (1) there would be greater continuity-of-care for the patient, (2) care would be more efficient, (3) outcomes recorded after a standard-of-care was used for a particular disease could be used to compare the standard-of-care with other standards of care for the disease, and (4) some care activities that are now done in the inpatient setting because they re-quire a team of coordinated caregivers could be done in the outpatient setting (e.g., outpatient surgery).

Unfortunately, chronic condition care today, especially in the United States, is treated as if it were acute care: there is little if any planning of long-term care and visits are often uncoordinated. A stay in a hospital does provide this coor-dination during the stay and perhaps for follow-up appointments, but remaining in a hospital when it is not necessary in order to coordinate care is extremely costly.

The reason that things do not go totally haywire today without this coordination between different physicians and other caregivers caring for the patient—and even lacking a complete medical record—is that there are "generally agreed-upon" standards of care for many diseases. However, differences in actual standards of care and lack of a complete patient medical record results in duplicate tests, lengthy interviews of the patient, and inefficient and costly care.

Even when there are no formalized teams (e.g., there are only independent physicians individually caring for a patient's chronic condition), team-based care techniques (e.g., planning care ahead of time) would enable better communication between physicians on the patient's condition and better continuity-of-care. In such a case, the physicians could then be viewed as a *virtual team.*

Over the life cycle of a disease process, there may be many *critical points* (Sackett et al. 1991) where a *critical point* is "a time before which therapy is more effective or easier to apply than afterwards." A physician or a team of physicians must be astute enough to look for and recognize critical points. Having a care plan based upon biomarkers for the condition could identify these critical points. Of particular concern is a medical condition that could change rapidly that has many critical points occurring within a short period of time.

Although team care and development of a case to track the patient's medical condition would most often be implemented upon diagnosis of a particular disease, a case may also be appropriate when a pre-disease condition is identified. For example, there are pre-cancerous tumors that may turn into cancer. Thus implementation of a case for a pre-disease condition that could result in the disease may be appropriate.

In order select the best standards of care, *outcomes* of a standard-of-care must be useful and well documented. Once standards of care for a particular medical condition are evaluated based upon evidence of effectiveness determined by outcomes and the best standards of care are chosen, new standards of care could be proposed and evaluated against the existing best standards of care. Standards of care should then be evaluated through clinical trials, where a *clinical trial* is "a formal method used to determine if a diagnostic, treatment or prevention measure is safe, effective, and better than a current standard-of-care." One method for a clinician to develop an initial care plan for a chronic condition is for the clinician to use narratives and diagrams in the national guideline database developed by the Agency for Healthcare Research (AHRQ) of the U.S. Department of Health & Human Resources, identifying evidence-based practice for chronic conditions. See reference (AHRQ 2006) for an example of such a guideline. Effective standards of care developed by the AHRQ in coordination with medical organizations could be put in a national guideline database for use by clinicians.

In summary, to support team-based care, whether it is actual teams or virtual teams, more precise standards of care are needed as well as a more team-friendly and patient-friendly patient medical record—a medical record that includes care plans based upon the standards of care that all clinicians would follow in the care of the patient. Outcomes of chosen standards of care should be clearly identified, and clinical trials to identify better or updated standards of care should be done to improve medicine.

2.2.3 Preventive Care

In the future there will be more preventive care to reduce the overall costs of medicine. Is it better to do preventive care for a disease or wait until the, possibly remote, possibility that the disease will occur and then try to cure the disease (Russell 1986)? Biomarkers such as age, sex, LDL cholesterol, blood pressure, genetics, and so on might identify an increased probability for a disease and thus may change the answer to this question for an individual. Whether or not a disease can be treated in its earlier phases could also change the answer.

In general, different types of preventive care may or may not be cost-effective, be worth the side effects, or be worth the chance of harm. For example, Pap smears for cervical cancer are relatively benign and generally cost-effective, at least for certain age groups of females. Prostate biopsies for prostate cancer may be unduly painful and sometimes may not be useful even when cancer is detected because many prostate cancers in men are slow growing, and treating them may cause more harm than good; on the other hand, such biopsies may be appropriate prior to a TURP to treat prostate enlargement, as the procedure could change upon the patient having prostate cancer. A recent journal article argues that guidelines for giving women mammograms should be reviewed as mammograms may result in the overtreatment of breast cancer as mammograms do not always distinguish low-risk cancers, which do not need to be immediately treated, from others (Esserman, Shieh, and Thompson 2009).

Many vaccinations—despite the publicity—have been shown to be cost-effective and cause harm only rarely, providing benefits that usually far outweigh their risks.

A patient medical record should be able to recommend and record vaccinations and worthwhile prevention interventions based upon medical industry guidelines and patient biomarkers. One way to record preventive health recommendations (such as vaccinations, Pap smears, PSA tests, mammograms, and colonoscopies) and inform a patient of a recommended intervention at the appropriate time is a *life care path*.

A *life care path* is "a clinical pathway identifying preventive care for an individual over a long period of time," where a *clinical pathway* is "a structured way to identify care activities and caregiver work flow needed to care for a patient with a particular condition or disease. Paths through a clinical pathway can be adjusted for the particular needs of an individual patient" (McGuire 2004).

2.2.4 Wellness

In the future, there will be a greater emphasis on wellness to reduce the costs of medicine. *Wellness* is the idea that healthy behaviors can increase longevity and protect against disease. Wellness can be thought of as a part of public health, as a way to save employers providing health insurance money, or as part of a comprehensive medical care system.

In the United States, wellness and also preventive care are most prominently promoted by *capitated* health care systems such as Health Maintenance Organizations (HMOs) where a fixed fee per month is paid for comprehensive health care, as preventing diseases rather than treating them when they are in an advanced stage could potentially save the HMO, as opposed to fee-for-service health care organizations, a significant amount of money. In HMOs wellness is promoted by their clinicians and HMO patient education programs.

Wellness is also promoted by some corporations to increase employee productivity and decrease medical insurance costs. For example, Warren Buffett, the Johnson and Johnson Corporation and others are trying to promote wellness, specifically wellness in the workplace (Campeau 2007).

Statistically, it has been determined that a change of lifestyles can promote health and longevity, including getting enough sleep and exercise, healthy eating and weight control, quitting smoking of cigarettes, getting dental care, and stress management.

For example, a condition known as "insulin resistance" that is clearly related to diet—and related to the chronic conditions of obesity, heart disease, type 2 diabetes, asthma, some cancers, and Alzheimer's disease—has become more prevalent in the United States since the 1970's. Type 2 diabetes afflicts 6% of adults, up from 3% in the 1970's. Obesity is up to 34% from 17% in the 1970's (Taubes 2009).

Mental health is also an important part of wellness. I propose that employees of large corporations be given a free initial mental health interview which could be combined with counseling on any job-related problems, as mental health problems could cause job-related problems and vice versa. I believe that this would save organizations money in that mental health problems are grossly undertreated and that together with job-related problems result in a large decrease in the productivity of employees. Such a mental health visit could be provided by a psychiatric clinical social worker, with the employee having the option of whether the visit would or would not be included in the individual's patient medical record. The psychiatric clinical social worker could recommend that the person come in for mental health care or could work as an ombudsman to direct the employee to resources in his company with whom the employee could consult to resolve job-related problems.

I predict that wellness will become a greater part of health care, particularly when wellness is not just understood statistically but is understood scientifically. I think that wellness will become better understood scientifically by a greater understanding of the workings of the brain.

Consider some of the following speculations about how wellness, the brain and disease interrelate:

Chronic stress and depression. Based upon the results of several scientific experiments, stress or depression could promote heart disease, stroke and a decrease in longevity. Using some of these studies, my hypothesis of how this happens is as follows: Adrenalin and subsequently cortisol are secreted into our blood streams when we are under stress. Secretion of cortisol and adrenalin are part of the "fight or flight" response which is initiated by the brain and shut off by the brain (if the body is working correctly, which it sometimes is not). When we are depressed or under continually occurring stress (such as being in a bad work situation), there is an over secretion of cortisol. Over secretion of cortisol is known to decrease the length of DNA (the ends of DNA called telomeres) when cells successively divide, and in that way is associated with decreased longevity (Stein 2004). When cortisol persists in the body for long period of time, it can attack blood vessels, setting off the body's immune system (Norden 2007); the immune system consequently causes inflammation of the blood vessels with the subsequent possible accumulation of plaque that could lead to both heart disease and stroke.

Chronic stress is also known to affect memory. It causes atrophy of the dendrites of neurons in the hippocampus of the brain, a part of the brain that plays a major role in long-term memory (Magrinos, Jose Verdugo, and McEwen 1997).

The endogenous reward system. Part of the brain affected by smoking, drugs, overindulgence in alcohol, and other addictive behaviors is called the "endogenous reward system" as it provides mental rewards for these behaviors. Over time, changes to other parts of the brain occur that make withdrawal even more difficult—for example, addiction affects the part of the frontal lobe of the prefrontal cortex that is involved in judgment and decision making (Norden 2007).

Touch and simulation and the brain. Touch and stimulation of infants has an effect on their brains. Infants who do not receive touch and simulation do not develop normally and later are more frightened of new situations and less trustful of other people (Colavita 2006). This has been shown by babies in orphanages in Romania who have not received stimulation from adults.

Knowing and thinking you know. Dr. Robert A. Burton in the book *On Being Certain: Believing You are Right Even When You're Not* contends that "knowledge" and "knowing what you know" are brain functions that occur in different parts of the brain and are not necessarily dependent upon each other (Burton 2008). A schizophrenic can know he is hearing voices from God, a person with bipolar disorder can know that he does not have that disease but instead everyone who thinks he does is wrong, and an ordinary person can be sure that he knows a particular item of knowledge even when he does not.

Violence in prisoners. A study has shown that prisoners given nutritional supplements committed 35% fewer violent incidents than those given a placebo. A follow-on study is currently being conducted (Bohannon 2009).

In the future, knowledge of how the brain functions could change how physicians treat patients, mothers raise children, the government treats drug addiction, and people in general evaluate their own opinions. In medicine in the future, there is likely to be a need for greater collaboration between physicians and clinicians who are experts on the brain in preventing and treating disease.

One difference between the brain and other organs (see figure 1) is that whereas most organs only have a limited number of different types of cells, there are many different types of neurons in the brain—according to a web site of the Canadian Institutes of Health Research there are over 200 different types of neurons in the brain (Canadian Institutes of Health Research 2002). Clearly there is a lot more to be learned about how the brain functions.

2.2.5 Patient Compliance and Patient Values

In the future, patients will be more involved in the care process. Patient care would be much easier if patients always complied with physician's dictates and orders, but they do not because of forgetfulness; work or family situations; lack of money; denial or fear; or the complexity of compliance, such as remembering to take medications at the right time and with the correct dosage.

In the future, patients could be assisted in complying with a physician's orders in the following ways:

- **Non-clinicians to advise the patient:** With team-care, there will be greater use of non-clinicians, including counselors and mental health personnel, to advise on life situations. There will be greater use of pharmacists to advise on medications and create schedules for the taking of multiple medications.

- **Patient-understandable written communication from clinicians:** Communication from a clinician with a patient after an encounter might be available on-line or on a print-out in layman's language including a physician's directives, prescriptions related to the patient's diseases, and future appointments.

- **Assistance in keeping appointments:** Future appointments will be available on-line or by phone. Reminder postcards will be sent to the patient and reminder phone calls would be made to the patient to help insure that the patient does not miss a visit. Patients could cancel and reschedule appointments on-line or by phone.

2.2.6 Multiple Medical Conditions

In the future, patient care that involves multiple medical conditions will be improved. Patient care would be much easier if medical conditions only occurred one at a time, but they often occur in combination, especially in the elderly. Multiple medical conditions occurring at the same time result in:

- Confusion in drug administration due to patients taking a greater number of drugs, resulting in errors in frequency or dosage.

- Greater possibility of drug interactions, again due to patients taking more medications.

- Greater complexity in standards of care due to the standards of care needing to address more than one disease.

- The need for triage of care, i.e., determining which medical condition should be treated first.

Consequently,

- There will be a need to assist patients who take many medications in the scheduling of the taking of their medications.
- There will be a need to identify drug interactions before drugs are prescribed.
- Standards of care for different medical conditions may need to be modified or merged to handle the multiple medical conditions effectively.
- There will be a need for more efficient use of clinicians who can triage care when care for some conditions must be given priority over others.

Triage is the assessment of patients' medical problems to determine urgency and priority of care to determine which patient is to be seen next, most often in the emergency department, or it is the assessment of a single patient's medical conditions to determine which ones should be given priority over the others. Consider a dramatic case of a single patient with multiple medical conditions requiring triage of care:

A man has a heart attack while driving causing him to run into a tree resulting in multiple injuries. Often a general surgeon would be assigned to the patient to determine the ordering of medical procedures to be performed as the patient will probably have to be stabilized for one medical condition before the other medical condition can be treated.

2.2.7 Other Changes

Health care will also be changing in the following ways in the future:

- **Payment based upon keeping patients healthy not only services provided:** Except for health care organizations such as Kaiser Permanente, the Mayo Clinic and other health care organizations where physicians are given fixed salaries and incentives for keeping patients healthy, payment of physicians in the United States is almost entirely based upon fee-for-service (i.e., upon the number of services provided). In entirely fee-for-service organizations there is a lesser incentive to keep patients healthy; to implement the best, most cost-effective, practices; to reduce medical errors; or to implement EPRs (or UPRs) that can track these activities and identify where costs can be saved. Medical payment methods will either change in the future from fee-for-service to salaried or implementation of EPRs (and UPRs) will continue to lag behind automation that occurs in other industries.

- **Digitized diagnostic imaging:** Diagnostic images such as x-rays, MRIs and CAT scans will become increasingly more digitized, being stored on computer files instead of on film. As a result, storage of diagnostic images will cost less, take up much less physical space and enable transferring of the image over a network to another clinician for care purposes or to a radiologist for interpretation (who could be located anywhere geographically). Transportation and analysis of a diagnostic image will cost less and use of successive diagnostic images to record and predict the progression of a medical condition will become more feasible.

- **The need for paper or scanned documents:** Even with automated EPR systems, there always will be a need for either paper medical records or medical record documents that are scanned. Examples are documents that need to be signed by the patient and thus need to display a signature such as advance directives or a consent form for medical or surgical procedures, and documents that can be taken home by the patient, filled out and returned. Scanned documents have the advantage over paper documents in that they can be displayed on-line.

- **Regenerative medicine and stem cells:** There is a potential for stem cells and non-stem cells to become replacement cells that could cure some diseases (e.g., a replacement bladder build from the patient's own cells (Smith 2006) or a transplant of pancreatic islet cells into the pancreas of a person with type I diabetes to restore insulin production (Ramiya et al. 2000)). Furthermore, stem cells could generate cells of various types that could be used to test the effects of a new drug on different cells of the body or to analyze a disease process (US Department of Health and Human Services 2006).

- **Other biological and technological innovations:** Innovations will range from synthetic biology and angiogenesis to new more powerful MRIs and mechanical assist devices. *Synthetic biology* is the application of genetic engineering to generate new biologic entities such as enzymes or vaccines or to redesign existing biological systems. *Angiogenesis* is the formation of new blood vessels that result from fast growing cells (such as cancer cells) sending out a signal to do so; one approach to fighting cancer is to stop growth of these blood vessels.

3

REQUIREMENTS AND DESIGN OF A UNIVERSAL PATIENT MEDICAL RECORD

This section modifies and greatly expands on information previously published in reference (McGuire 2006).

Medical institutions and single physicians have or will be implementing electronic patient record (EPR) systems to automate their medical records. A universal patient medical record (UPR) would provide a means of combining medical information from these EPR systems and would enable medical support services that could only be properly performed by looking at the total of the patient's health information (e.g., drug-drug interaction detection and management of patient care that could occur in different medical organizations with different EPR systems).

A UPR would be a *distributed* patient medical record (i.e., stored in many different locations) that summarizes and electronically combines all of a patient's medical information and would be available to all clinicians caring for the patient no matter where the clinician or patient is located in the world (McGuire 2004). This section will identify the following:

- How a UPR could make improvements to health care
- How I propose a UPR should be structured to make these improvements

- How an electronic patient record system (EPR) could be changed to incorporate such a UPR.

3.1 How a UPR Could Improve Health Care

A UPR could potentially improve health care in the following ways:

- **Complete medical record:** It can provide a complete (longitudinal) patient medical record.
- **Past medical history:** It can provide an always-available past medical history for a patient, even when the patient shows up in a health care institution where the patient has not been seen before.
- **Public health:** It can improve public health and make public health a greater part of medical care.
- **Medical condition management:** It can help support overall management of a patient's chronic conditions and support management of episodes of care (time periods of intense care for a medical condition), thus providing better continuity-of-care. As part of this process, intermediate and long-term outcomes could be recorded, enabling the care of the patient to be evaluated. Care for one medical condition could take into consideration a patient's other medical conditions.
- **Patient information related to overall care:** It can record important patient medical information not related to any one encounter such as advance directives and biomarkers that can be used to predict disease.
- **Patient compliance:** Through the UPR, the clinician could provide information to the patient to fa-

cilitate patient compliance with physician directives and orders.

- **Makes care more transparent and supports accountability.** (Note: In the pay for service world this may be considered a liability.)

- **Referrals and consultations:** It would enable a primary care physician to refer a patient to a specialty physician with transfer of the referral request to the specialty physician. It would enable a primary care physician to request or record a consultation with a specialty physician with transfer of the consultation response back to the primary care physician. With telecommunications it could support multiple providers caring for the patient, with providers remotely located from each other or from the patient.

- **Drug interactions and other alerts:** With the complete past medical history, it would enable a physician to be alerted when a patient with an allergy comes in, when a medication order could result in a drug interaction, or when an order could result in a duplicate order. It would enable a specialist physician to be alerted upon a patient referral or consultation request or a primary care physician upon a consultation response or the completion of a referral.

- **Research:** It can support research.

- **Money:** It can save money.

3.1.1 Complete Medical Record

The UPR could provide a complete medical record for the patient. Consider an example of the medical records for a female member of a large HMO (see figure 4):

The HMO member was almost always seen within the HMO. The HMO member, however, had visits outside the HMO prior to joining the HMO. There are a number of non-HMO health care organizations allied with the HMO; this HMO member had a baby at one of these alliance health care organizations, paid for by the HMO.

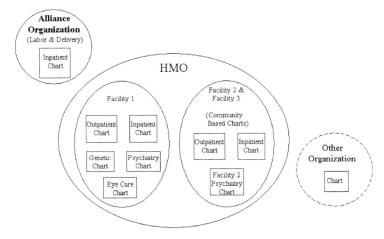

Figure 4 Example of a patient's medical records.

If the HMO automated their medical records with an EPR system, then the member's medical records within the HMO would be available via automation to any HMO clinician seeing the patient. Medical records from organizations outside but allied with the HMO may or may not also be available on the same EPR system.

Medical records in other organizations would not be available through the HMO's EPR system. A universal patient medical record would make *all* the medical records—either inside or outside the HMO—immediately available to an HMO clinician and to all authorized clinicians outside the HMO also.

Figure 4, however, shows the most ideal situation for availability of medical records for a patient, where the patient is seen primarily in a single health care organization, an HMO. Many patients in the United States are seen in many different unaffiliated health care organizations and thus a universal patient medical record is even more beneficial for such patients.

In order to combine medical records from many different EPR systems, I propose that the universal patient medical record (UPR) system—see figure 5—record every patient encounter (e.g., outpatient visit, inpatient stay, procedure visit, emergency department visit).

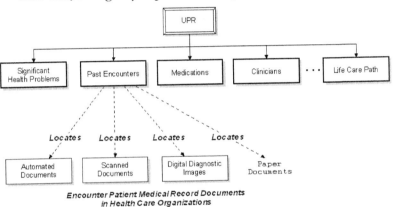

Encounter Patient Medical Record Documents
in Health Care Organizations

Figure 5 UPR provides a medical history and a complete medical record.

For each encounter, the UPR would include the clinician(s) seen, the date of the encounter, the location of the encounter, the diagnoses, the names of the encounter medical record documents, and locators of each of the documents in EPR systems. The information on an encounter and locators of the encounter medical records could come from an EPR system during or after a patient encounter.

After it is created, the encounter information in the UPR could be displayed to a clinician in the form of a "Clinical Summary" for a patient, for example, as shown in figure 6. A list of the past encounters for the patient would be displayed. A clinician could select an encounter and then select one of the medical records created during the encounter for display after retrieval of the medical record from the EPR system where it is located. (Note that in the example, UPHN stands for the "universal patient health number" (ASTM 2009), a patient identifier that is unique to the patient.)

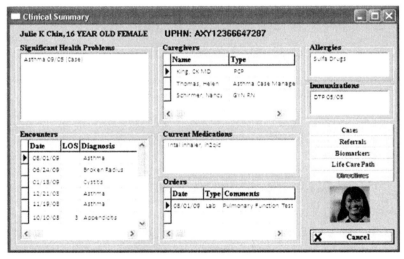

Figure 6 Example of a past medical history developed from the UPR.

A medical record document for an encounter could be an EPR-stored automated medical record document, scanned document, or digital diagnostic image, in which case such a document could potentially be retrieved from the

EPR system upon clinician selection of the encounter and named document, or the document could be a medical record document stored in a chart room, in which case it could be ordered from the health care organization where it was created upon clinician selection of the encounter and named document. I assume that the medical record document retrieved from an EPR system and displayed through the UPR would contain data in the form it was entered at the health care organization using data formats used at the health care organization, whereas the Clinical Summary would use industry-agreed upon data formats.

3.1.2 An Always-Available Past Medical History

The UPR could provide a complete, always-available past medical history for the patient.

Some people advocate that patients keep their own patient-maintained past medical history on-line on the Internet. Such a patient medical history is called a *personal health record*.

I propose that a past medical history be developed from medical information sent from the EPR systems to the UPR, or otherwise from medical information input and updated by clinicians and patients from corrections of UPR information. Such an approach would likely produce a past history that is more accurate and up-to-date than the personal health record.

With a UPR, if a patient shows up in a health care organization anywhere in the world and can be identified by smart card, biometric or other identification—even if the patient was unconscious—the clinician would have a complete past medical history for the patient. The past medical history could include significant health problems, allergies and medications and could potentially save the patient's life.

I propose that such a past medical history include:

- Significant health problems (with the clinician option of viewing past retired significant health problems)
- Encounters with drill-down to medical documents
- Current medications (with the option of viewing all ordered medications)
- Current clinicians (with the option of viewing all clinicians)
- Recent orders
- Allergies
- Etc.

An example past medical history for a patient—here called a "Clinical Summary"—appears in figure 6. Through the Clinical Summary, the clinician would be able to view information in the UPR (see figure 5). And as noted earlier, by selecting an encounter, the clinician could list the names of medical record documents for the encounter and drill down to an automated or scanned medical document or diagnostic digital image to display.

Most of the information in the UPR would be automatically updated from information in EPRs. Some information might be input or modified by clinicians or patients. The rules for creating and modifying particular information must be agreed upon by the medical community and system designers. Examples of possible rules are the following:

- **Encounters:** Encounters and encounter medical document names and locations would be automatically sent to the UPR by an EPR system. At the end of an encounter, a clinician without an EPR system might be able to enter the encounter directly in the UPR.

- **Medications:** All prescribed medications would be sent by the EPR system as a result of clinician orders through the EPR system or entered by the clinician through the UPR after the encounter. A clinician could identify that a medication is a current medication and/or identify how long it would be a current medication. A clinician could identify that a medication was no longer being taken by the patient.

- **Recent outstanding orders:** Orders would be sent down by the EPR system or, for the case of no EPR, the clinician could enter them at the end of the encounter. When an EPR system indicates the order was filled then it would be removed. A clinician could remove an order, indicating it was filled or entered by mistake. The UPR might be notified of the order fulfillment by the EPR system from an ancillary system (e.g., a clinical laboratory system connected to the EPR system could indicate that all clinical lab results have been received with the EPR system sending informing the UPR to remove the order).

- **Significant health problems:** A clinician could add to a list of the patient's significant health problems, or indicate which ones no longer apply or were entered incorrectly. A patient could add a significant health problem or indicate it no longer applies, with clinicians later verifying the correctness of the information.

At the beginning and end of a visit, the clinician may be able to do an overall verification and update of patient medical information in the UPR. An audit trail of changes should be kept.

3.1.3 Public Health a Greater Part of Medicine

In the twentieth century, life span increased approximately 30 years. Most of this increase was due to public health rather than medical care (Farmer and Lawrenson 2004). Although some of these public health measures such as cleaner drinking water and air and more abundant food are outside of medicine, some public health measures that have increased life spans are a part of medicine:

- Immunizations (e.g., for tetanus, influenza)
- Diagnostic tests for purposes of disease control (e.g., a test for a type of pandemic influenza, TB, HIV/AIDS and malaria)
- Diagnostic tests for purposes of prevention (e.g., colonoscopies, mammograms, PSA tests).

Immunizations and preventive health tests can be tracked in the UPR for each patient. They can be scheduled via life care paths, where again a *life care path* is "a clinical pathway identifying preventive care for an individual over a long period of time, scheduling preventive care based upon criteria such as age, sex, past medical history." Through the life care path, either the patient could be informed to call in to schedule a preventive care activity, or the patient could be automatically scheduled for the care activity (e.g., a mammogram). In general, a life care path would be managed by the patient's primary care physician.

The UPR could automatically send patient disease information to public health organizations and other disease registries when it detects reportable health care events. In particular, the UPR could report on nosocomial infections and other medically cased illnesses to government or health care agencies; such agencies could also search the UPR to identify unreported medically caused illnesses.

Through the UPR, public health agencies can do epidemiological studies removing identification of the patients. For example, the sperm count of men throughout the world decreased 50% in 50 years (Carlsen et al. 1992); through the UPR, public health agencies, using sperm count as a biomarker, could identify which geographic areas had men with higher and lower sperm counts, and then potentially identify environmental causes.

Public health agencies can quickly determine if an influenza or other vaccine is causing health problems by tracking the patients who have been given a new vaccine and identify which ones do and do not have pre-existing conditions.

When a disease outbreak is detected in a geographic location without the necessary number of clinicians, the UPR could enable a clinician to consult on the care of patients located remotely from the clinician, where patients are in a remote location of the United States or the world, or where the clinician is a type of specialist not locally available.

3.1.4 Management of Medical Conditions

Chronic conditions (e.g., asthma, epilepsy) account for over 70 percent each of outpatient visits, inpatient stays, and prescriptions (Partnership for Solutions et al. 2002). David Lawrence, MD, the former CEO of Kaiser Permanente, in his book *From CHAOS to CARE* recommended having team-based care for chronic conditions to improve continuity-of-care (Lawrence 2003); this team approach to chronic condition care would make medical care more efficient and less costly at the same time as it would likely improve patient care.

A *case* is "an organized (automated or non-automated) system for managing the delivery of health care to an individual for a medical condition or conditions that includes assessment and development of a plan of care, coordination of services, referrals and follow-ups"(McGuire 2004). The purpose of a case is to allow a physician to take time and preplan how clinicians will provide care over time and to allow care to be consistently provided even when the physician is unavailable. Because of preplanning and consistent care, the total time for care would likely be less than if there was no preplanning.

Case management documents along with health care organizations functioning differently than they do now could support this team-based care. The case document would include a care plan for the chronic condition developed by the principal clinician. The care plan would be followed by subsequent clinicians to insure consistency of care. Encounters dealing with the chronic condition would be identified in the case with care given based upon the care plan or deviating from the care plan with encounter medical documents explaining any deviations.

In order to account for second opinions and other consultations that might change the case care plan, these consultations (e.g., possibly identifying improved treatments) would also be included with the care documentation. The principal clinician together with the patient could then optionally incorporate these ideas in a revised care plan. The care plan could be modified or redone with clear explanations of why the care plan changed.

A case could also record intermediate outcomes and long-term outcomes, where an outcome is a "measurement of the value of a particular course of therapy." Recording outcomes would enable the results of patient care to be evaluated and would enable the course of therapy to be compared with alternative ones.

Figure 7 identifies one way to store and locate case documentation through use of a UPR. For each patient, information on each case for the patient (e.g., a case dealing with chronic care of asthma) would be stored in the UPR. A clinician could identify a new case, optionally associating it with a significant health problem. The clinician could identify the case manager and case team members then or later.

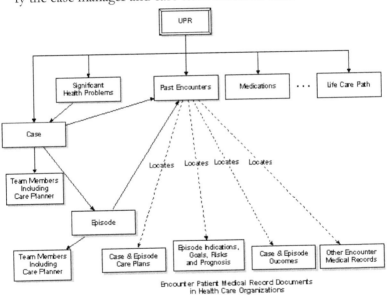

Figure 7 UPR information for a case.

When an encounter occurs that is related to an existing case (e.g., an outpatient visit for asthma), the clinician could identify that the encounter relates to an existing case. The clinician should follow any existing case care plan. Other medical records created during the encounter would be automatically associated with the case via being associated with the encounter associated with the case.

Besides use of a case for an existing chronic condition, a case could be developed for a pre-disease condition that may potentially turn into a disease. For example, if colon polyps were detected and removed during a colonoscopy, then a case might be opened to track the patient over the patient's life time for possible development of future polyps or development of colon cancer.

In the possible progression of a disease (see figure 8), there are often critical points, where a *critical point* (Sackett et al. 1991) is "a time before which therapy is more effective or easier to apply than afterwards." A clinician may wish to set up a case to remind the clinician and patient to beware of such critical points occurring. Again in our example, when polyps are found during the colonoscopy, the clinician might use the case to schedule future colonoscopies to check for further polyps and insure that a critical point of a polyp turning into colon cancer is not reached.

Besides being created for disease management, a case could be created for other purposes. Examples are cases for a worker compensation care or for tracking the overall care of a Medicare patient who frequently moves between health care institutions (e.g., outpatient care, inpatient care in a hospital, inpatient care in a SNF, care at home, and inpatient care in a nursing home).

It is expected that during the time that a case tracks a chronic condition, disease process or possible pre-disease situation, there will likely be periods of intense team-based care, which I will term *episodes of care* that will occur as part of the case. An episode of care would be treated much like a case with its own care plan and outcomes. For example, a life-long case could be set up for a person who had just received a severe knee injury. The initial episode of care might be the initial knee surgery and rehabilitation period, a

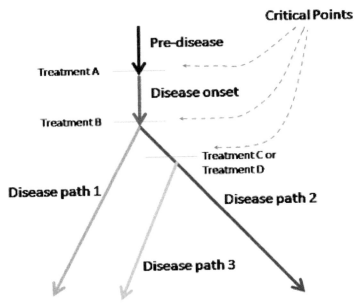

Figure 8 Disease progression map.

later episode might be taking out the pin that was put in the knee, and a much later episode might be a knee replacement, with each episode recording a final outcome for the episode. In the intervening periods, the patient might receive less intense care such as being given advice and medication for osteoarthritis and advice on when, if ever, to schedule re-placement surgery. A critical point might occur when the patient's osteoarthritis gets so bad that the patient requires a strong narcotic to control pain and has the potential of becoming addicted; a knee replacement might be a better choice.

In general, a case would be managed by the patient's primary care physician, while an episode would be managed by a specialist physician and overseen by the primary care physician. In order to provide a check on quality of care for an episode of care, upon seeing a patient after an episode of care by a specialty physician, a primary care physician could provide an independent outcome of the episode of care within the case or the episode.

See figure 7 again. Each episode could be assigned an episode team manager. Like for the case, encounters, care plans and outcomes could be associated with the episode. It is expected that payments for specialist care would more commonly be based upon an episode rather than the case, even perhaps with the payment partially determined by the episode outcome; thus payment would be made for an entire episode of care, whereas payment for the long-term, ongoing case would otherwise be made for each encounter. An episode care plan is likely to be more detailed than the corresponding part of the case care plan and probably more health care organization specific. Through episode care plans without the identities of patients, health care organizations could share ideas on best practices and ideas on processes to avoid medical mistakes.

Provided to the patient at the start of an episode of care, the physician would identify the indications (i.e., criteria) for a patient to receive the treatment, the goals of the episode, risks of the treatment and what will be done to avoid these risks, and the prognosis for the patient at the end of the episode (i.e., the expected outcomes). For example, for a total knee replacement, the indications for the patient to receive the treatment might be that "severe osteoarthritis where conservative treatments have been exhausted." The goals of the knee replacement might be "greatly decreased pain in the knee with normal function of the knee." The risks in receiving the treatment include "deep vein thrombosis, fractures, loss of motion, instability and infection." And the prognosis for the patient after the episode might be "achievement of all the goals with the avoidance of all risks" (Wikipedia 2009).

In order to promote continuity-of-care, the case or episode care plan should be the responsibility of one clinician with inclusion of any changes in the care plan due to second opinions entered by that clinician. If the patient is dissatisfied with the care given, the patient could give permission to transfer this duty to another clinician.

When a patient has multiple chronic conditions, there is likely to be multiple cases, episodes and care plans. The clinicians doing the respective care plans should consult with each other to identify when each care plan should address co-morbidities.

Like for a life care path, a case or episode could, at the appropriate time, send the patient a request to call in to schedule a case or episode care activity, or, alternatively, the case or episode could automatically schedule the care activity. For example, a case for a patient with type I diabetes could have the patient come in periodically to have an eye test and to have the patient's cholesterol checked in addition to other health checks for the diabetes; if the patient with diabetes had the complication of foot problems, an episode or another case could be opened that has a care plan that schedules care activities to diagnose and treat diabetes foot problems (Neighmond 2008).

3.1.5 Patient Information Related to Overall Care

Medical information that is related to the patient and overall care rather than any one encounter is the following that could also be included in the UPR—see figure 9:

- **Patient directives:** Examples are advance directives, organ and tissue donor directives, and patient agreement to allow patient information via email and on the Internet.
- **Overall and disease-related biomarkers:** Genomic information and other biomarkers.
- **Disease progression map associated with a significant health problem:** A diagram to identify the progression of a disease over time and current status of the patient in the disease progression, identifying critical points in the progression of the disease (McGuire 2004). See figure 8.

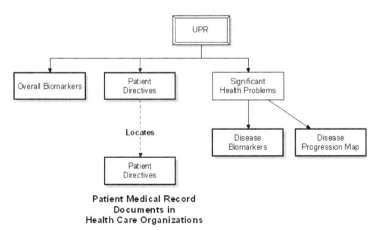

Figure 9 Non-encounter information about the patient.

Advance directives are "instructions from a patient, most often at the time of admission to a hospital, informing medical personnel of the patient's wishes for treatments and care. Advance directives only apply when the patient is incapacitated and enable to make decisions for herself or himself." For example, the advance directive might identify who is to make decisions for you when you are enable to yourself and may identify to "not resuscitate" under certain conditions. Advance directives may not apply in certain situations; for example, during and after an operation, the surgeon may take all extraordinary measures to keep the patient alive despite what is in the advance directive. (Note: Storage of an advance directive in the UPR may open up the potential of the advance directive being applicable for all hospital stays rather than just the current one, with the patient being able to change the advance directives at any time.)

Biomarkers are "cellular, biochemical, molecular, or genetic characteristics or alterations by which a normal, abnormal, or simply biologic process can be recognized, or monitored" (NIH 2000). The genome of an individual is a fixed biomarker, while other biomarkers may change over time (e.g., blood pressures, PSA, mammograms, etc.) In the future, genomic information may become more important in medical care. If it does, it would then make sense to save this information once in the UPR rather than in any one EPR system, as genomic information will always be costly to determine.

Some biomarkers are related to the overall health status of the patient (e.g., the genome, blood pressure), while others may be related to a specific disease (e.g., the PSA for BPH and prostate cancer, or the genetic characteristics of a type of liver cancer). The former type of non-disease specific biomarker I call an *overall biomarker*. The latter I call a *disease biomarker*, and I suggest it be associated with a significant health problem. Associating a disease biomarker with a case is another possibility.

Overall and disease biomarkers could be recorded over time and produce a graph (e.g., PSA values over time) to identify disease progression. In the future, one biomarker could be a diagnostic digital image located within an EPR system with a series of diagnostic images for the same body system (e.g. of the same knee) identifying disease progression of that body system over time. (Note that, unlike other biomarkers, the diagnostic images would not be stored in the UPR but would be stored in one or more EPR systems.)

Through the tracking of chronic conditions with use of cases, disease biomarkers, and disease progression maps, prognoses for diseases will become more accurate. This will include a greater accuracy in predicting end of life situations.

As a consequence of better prediction of end of life situations, there will be fewer "heroic" treatments that have a remote possibility of extending life at the expense of misery to the patient. Consequently, there will an even greater use of *hospice (palliative) care*, treatment (usually provided at the end of a patient's life) to relieve the symptoms of a disease to make the patient more comfortable rather than to provide a cure. Some experts have advocated the greater use of hospice care for patients with severe dementia who meet certain criteria that indicate that their dementia has reached an end of life condition (Mitchell et al. 2009).

And instead of care in the ICU (Intensive Care Unit) that may extend a patient's life by heroic means with decreased quality of life, a patient should have the choice of in-the-hospital "comfort" care or home care instead, as being a human pin cushion and being without sleep in the ICU in one's remaining days is neither a pleasant experience for the patient or the patient's family.

3.1.6 Information for the Patient

In order to facilitate patient compliance with clinician directives and orders, I propose that the following be available to patients on-line on the Internet from information in the universal patient medical record—see figure 10:

- A list of past encounters with drill-down to medical records for a recent encounter, including clinical laboratory reports.
- For each encounter, clinician dictates to the patient using the language of the patient.
- For each episode, indications for a patient to have the treatment, goals of the episode, risks of treatment, and the prognosis for the patient after the episode. (This information should be available to the patient prior to the start of the episode.)
- Significant health problems of the patient.
- For a significant health problem, clinician dictates to the patient for the health problem using the language of the patient.
- Outstanding orders and referrals. (Note: if the patient needs to contact a clinician or other person for a referral, this contact information would be available here.)
- Current patient medications.
- Future appointments.
- The patient's current clinicians and their email addresses.

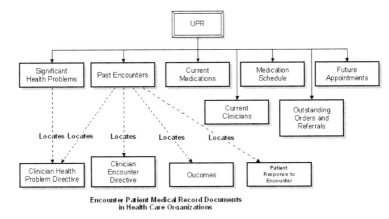

Figure 10 Information for the patient.

A patient should be able to respond to information in the UPR including information in encounter medical records and encounter and health problem directives to the patient from the clinician. The Health Insurance Privacy and Accountability Act (HIPAA) stipulates that patients must be permitted to review and amend their medical records.

3.1.7 Transparency and Accountability

With a UPR, there would be more transparency: the actions of clinicians and patients would be more obvious to patients, other clinicians caring for the patient and regulatory agencies through the documentation available in the UPR. For an episode, the patient would be informed by the physician of the indications for treatment, goals of treatment, risks of treatment, and prognosis (expected outcomes) prior to the episode. Clinicians and regulatory agencies would be able to more easily identify inconsistencies in the care of the patient by clinicians, whether an inconsistency was due to clinician error, disagreements or fraud. Also patient abuse of medical care would be more transparent to clinicians: a clinician would be alerted of a patient request for a duplicate prescription for a narcotic which could identify addictive behavior.

As stated earlier, HIPAA stipulates that patients must be permitted to review and amend their medical records (Department of Health and Human Services 2000). Through the EPR and from the UPR, patients could review their medical records and past medical history and add amendments to their medical record. In particular, patients would have access to instructions from the clinician for the patient related to significant health problems or related to an encounter and respond to each of these. The patient could verify that the care recorded in the medical record was indeed given to the patient. I propose that patients have a fixed period of time after an encounter to respond to what happened during the encounter and respond to what was recorded in the medial record, enabling the clinician to respond to and learn from the patient's input while the clinician still remembers all details of the visit.

The patient and clinician should both be able to report on adverse events through the UPR, including adverse reactions to vaccinations or medicine, procedures that caused harm, nosocomial infections (infections that occurred in a hospital), or injuries caused by a consumer product. These events could be reported to the health care organization, payers, the FDA, the Consumer Product Safety Commission, medical device manufacturers, or pharmaceutical companies.

Clinician transparency promotes clinician accountability. For instance, from reliable sources I learned that at one HMO when a scheduling system was implemented that recorded a physician's total time (seeing outpatients and inpatients as well as other non-patient time) that some physicians who were previously misreporting time quit the HMO. These physicians were suddenly forced to be accountable.

3.1.8 Referrals and Consultations

Through the universal patient medical record, a primary care physician could make a referral request for a patient to a specialty physician with a referral response being returned by the specialty physician upon the patient being seen. Also, the primary care physician can make a request for a consultation where the patient is not seen by the specialty physician, with the consultation response being returned by the specialty physician to the primary care physician. Both physicians would have access to the patient's medical history and the patient's medical documents at the same time through the UPR. Referral requests, consultation requests, referral responses and consultation responses could all be transferred between physicians through the UPR. (Note that a large health care organization with its own EPR system might want to handle internal—i.e., inside the health care organization—referrals and consults through its EPR system, but handle outside referrals and consults through the UPR.)

The UPR could also potentially support real-time consultations (e.g., through telecommunications—telephone or video—or face-to-face). Both physicians would have access to the patient's medical history and the patient's medical documents through the UPR. With simultaneous access to the patient's medical record, the specialty provider could be entering the consultation response while the primary care physician is seeing the patient and also updating the patient's medical record.

Also triage of a patient's medical problems could be done through telecommunications with a general surgeon or other physician consulting on the triage located remotely from the patient.

3.1.9 Alerts to Physicians Upon Medical Concerns

With the previous recording of a patient's allergies in the past medical history of the universal patient medical record, a physician could be alerted when a patient with an allergy comes in for care. Further, with the previous recording of a patient's medications, a physician's medication order for the patient could be checked against medications in the UPR for drug-drug interactions and drug allergies. With the UPR enabling transfer of referral requests, consultation requests, and consultation responses, a specialist physician could be alerted upon a patient referral or consultation request being received, and a primary care physician could be alerted upon a consultation response being returned.

3.1.10 Research and Comparative Effectiveness Analysis

Clinical and medical research and epidemiological studies could be supported by transferring information in the UPR to a data warehouse—a large database—with removal of patients' identities from the data. For example, a study could be done of the genetic similarity of patients encountering a particular side effect of a medication.

Removing information that can be used to identify a patient (*protected health information*) from medical records to create information for medical research is a concept introduced by HIPAA called *de-identification* (University of Wisconsin-Madison 2003).

Using information from cases and episodes of care in the UPR, the comparative effectiveness of treatment options and standards of care could be determined based upon outcomes recorded in the cases and episodes.

(Note that the evaluation of treatments simply based upon outcomes may sometimes be very difficult. For example, at this time, psoriasis can be controlled but cannot be cured. Treatments could include ultraviolet light therapy in the medical office twice a week or using a medication that requires a blood test at least every month. Whether such treatments that cannot provide a cure have benefits that exceed the time required for the treatments or the downside of having to take constant blood tests is individualized to the patient and the patient's life situation.)

Autopsy information could also be put in the UPR. This would enable researchers to evaluate the accuracy of diagnoses and the effectiveness of medical treatment.

3.1.11 Saving Money

By providing medical information collected over multiple encounters at all health care organizations where the patient was seen, the universal patient medical record would make a clinician's time more productive. Instead of creating a past medical history from scratch each time the patient comes in for care, the clinician could simply verify and update the existing past medical history in the UPR. Instead of creating a new care plan for a patient with a chronic condition, the clinician could use an existing care plan contained in case documentation for the chronic condition from the UPR. Medicare and Worker's Compensation patients could be more easily tracked. Referrals and consultations could also be speeded up, as noted earlier.

Upon a clinician order or prescription through the EPR, the EPR could request the UPR to check for duplicate diagnostic tests or prescriptions, saving the cost of duplicate tests or prescriptions. Through the UPR, payers could more easily check for billing inconsistent with care, detecting input errors and fraud.

Essential patient information such as advance directives, organ and tissue donation directives, or costly-to-determine genomic information could be recorded once in the UPR instead of many times in possibly unknown locations in the patient medical record, and thus be less costly to find and maintain. Preventive care tests could be more easily tracked and scheduled, and disease could then be caught at an earlier stage when it is easier and less costly to treat.

With patient care being more transparent, clinicians and regulatory agencies could more easily recognize when least-cost care for the best outcomes was not being followed. Through on-line patient instructions after a visit, a patient would more likely comply with the clinician's dictates, which could decrease the number of times the patient would need to come in for further care.

Government reimbursements for medical care could be decreased by the government requiring that clinicians follow evidence-based medicine (best practices); and requiring that clinicians generally prescribe less costly generic drugs instead of brand name drugs. The government could refuse to pay for nosocomial infections (infections acquired in the hospital) and medically caused errors—made more obvious through a UPR—which would require health organizations to improve its health care practices, saving money. (Note: An article in *JAMA* states that medical errors may be the third leading cause of death in the United States (Starfield 2000)).

By clinician and patient reporting of vaccination and medicine adverse events, pharmaceutical companies and the FDA could more quickly identify vaccinations and medicines that are causing harm and more quickly restrict their use, saving costs in extra medical care.

Enforcement of best practices by use of a universal patient medical record can be facilitated by cases and episodes. Use of the case structure enables care for a chronic condition to be tracked over a long period of time, and enables evaluation of care plans by comparing care plans against recorded outcomes of care. Because a case may occur over a long period of time, it might be useful, especially for specialty payment purposes, to break parts of cases up into episodes of care, periods of time during the case where intensive care occurs, such as a surgery (see figure 7). At the end of the episode an outcome of the episode could be determined. The payment for an episode could be based both on services provided and episode outcome. Also to make reimbursement fair, such reimbursement might also be based upon the *acuity* of the patient, i.e., upon the relative health of the patient, with more money paid for an unhealthy patient—this is to not penalize clinicians who accept sicker patients. Payment for episodes based on outcomes could save money by rewarding quality care.

3.2 Building the UPR from EPR Systems

The information in the UPR system would be created from information sent to it by EPR systems. Information could either be a by-product of normal operations of the EPR system, additional information entered by the clinician through the EPR or Internet, or information entered by the patient, possibly through the EPR system via the Internet. Current EPR systems would largely remain the same but require some internal modifications and some additional subsystems.

The EPR could use its current data standards, but should be able to convert some of its data to agreed-upon UPR data standards if the EPR data standards differ. For example, a British EPR system using Read codes might need to convert some Read codes to ICD for diagnoses and CPT for procedures for the Read code information to be used by the UPR.

One data element in the UPR might be a "universal patient health number," which could be a unique identifying number for the patient independent of health care organization. In such a case, there would be the need for an "assigning authority" to assign such a unique number to a patient or to look up and verify the patient's number, which could come from a "smart card". One approach that might obviate the need for a patient to carry identification is to use *biometrics*, identifying a person based up measurable biological characteristics such as voice, fingerprints, palm print, signature, or other means. The local medical record number in an EPR system medical record would have to be replaced with the universal patient health number when clinical information is sent to the UPR.

(Note that the country of Taiwan healthcare system carries this smart card approach one step further. It puts the whole past medical history for a patient on a smart card carried by the patient, with everyone's medical history also kept on a central database (Adams 2009).)

3.2.1 Proposed Network for EPRs and UPR
Proposed is that the universal patient medical record (UPR) be made available to any EPR system via a secure health care network. See figure 11.

This paper assumes that large health care organizations would want to use their own EPR systems, while small health care organizations may want to contract for outside EPR system services. In the latter case, the company owning the EPR system would serve similarly to a utility (e.g., a water or electrical company) providing service with costs based upon how often the service was used.

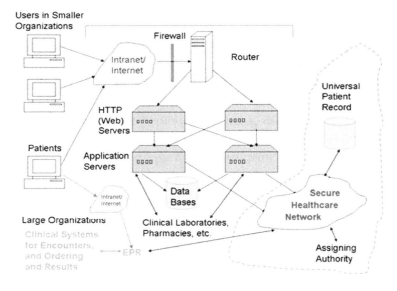

Figure 11 A secure health care network to connect EPR and UPR systems.

A large health care organization with its own clinical laboratories, pharmacies, etc. and associated clinical systems would likely interface its clinical systems directly with its health care organization EPR system and provide access to patients to EPR and UPR information through the Internet or an Intranet connected to the EPR system. The EPR system would communicate with the UPR through the secure health care network. The EPR system would send a limited amount of medical record information to the UPR including orders and sent orders to other clinical systems (pharmacy, clinical lab, etc.) for fulfillment. The other clinical systems could send back clinical laboratory, radiology and other results to the EPR that the EPR would also send to the UPR. Besides the clinical systems that handled orders (the clinical laboratory, pharmacy, radiology systems, etc.), there would be clinical systems for encounters that interface with the EPR system including hospital admission systems (for admissions, discharges and transfers), a scheduling system (for scheduling appointments), and a registration system (for registering the patient when the patient shows up for an outpatient visit); the EPR system would in turn sent encounter information to the UPR.

Smaller health care organizations could have access to an EPR system via an applications service provider (ASP). An ASP would provide EPR services via an Intranet to the health care organization—which may be referred to as "utility computing" as such an ASP may charge the health care organization for use of the ASP as an electrical utility might (Birman and Ritsko 2004). The ASP might have a large number of contracts with clinical laboratories and other ancillary systems to pass orders and receive results (or might in the future instead have access to these systems via the UPR). The EPR system would access the UPR through the secure health care network. Again, the EPR system would provide patient access to EPR and UPR information via the Internet or an Intranet through the EPR system.

Directly after a visit with a clinician, the patient should have access to his or her past medical history and visit medical records, including any clinician instructions for the visit. The patient should have the ability to add amendments to correct or comment on encounter medical record documents, with this information being sent back to the clinician via the EPR system. The patient should also have the ability to record any of the patient's adverse reactions to medications, vaccinations or procedures, or the patient receiving any nosocomial infections. This access should be over the Internet at home, or should be over an Intranet at the health care organization.

(One relatively secure approach to enable a patient to view the patient's UPR information at home after an encounter, including the medical records for the encounter, is for the patient to be emailed a link to this information together with a password that the patient must enter to view it and enter comments. As an option or for a patient who does not want to use the Internet, the patient could receive the information via mail or directly after a visit, allowing the patient to review it and return written comments.)

In the future there will likely be many UPRs that would each handle a subset of patients with the need for communication between the UPRs.

3.2.2 UPR Data from EPR Medical Record Documents

For ethical and legal reasons, an electronic patient record system (EPR) needs to produce medical record documents from clinical information entered in the EPR when recording the care activities for patients—this is true even when the EPR allows a clinician to enter clinical information from a computer screen that does not match the format of a medical record document. Much of the universal patient medical record (UPR) can be created from the collective EPR medical record documents. In the proposed design, the UPR can display all medical record documents except those that are non-automated and stored in chart rooms.

There are four types of medical record documents:

- **Automated medical record forms:** medical record forms created from clinical information entered through an EPR system.
- **Scanned medical record forms:** scanned paper medical record forms that are given digitized *index* data to allow the scanned form to be retrieved and displayed in the EPR or UPR systems.
- **Diagnostic digital images:** an image from an x-ray, MRI or other medical device used for diagnosis that is recorded in numerical form so it can be stored on a computer.
- **Chart room medical records:** paper medical records or non-digitized diagnostic images such as x-rays on film.

Challenges in using EPR medical record documents to partially create the UPR and to display the medical records through the UPR are many fold:

- Some types of medical record forms used by different health care organizations are similar but not necessarily the same (e.g., a history and physical).
- Some types of medical record forms are unique to a health care organization or differ markedly from one health care organization to another.
- Data used for the same purpose in EPR medical record documents and the UPR may have a different formats (e.g., a local medical record number in an EPR vs. a universal patient health number in the UPR). Using industry-agreed upon data formats in the UPR would enable medical records from differ-

ent health care organizations and thus different EPR systems to be organized for display through the UPR (e.g., having the same format patient, encounter, case and episode identifiers).

- When an EPR medical record document is displayed through the UPR, a clinician probably would want to see the clinical information as the clinician entered it. This information could use a data format only used at the health organization where the data was entered and may even be in a different language than used by the UPR.

- It is inefficient to redundantly store EPR medical records in the UPR, so a method of retrieval of a document for display in the UPR from EPR systems should be provided.

3.2.2.1 Use of XML

An emerging standard for storing medical record documents in an automated system is XML (e.g., HL7 XML Clinical Document Architecture, CDA (Dolin et al. 2001)). I propose that each automated medical record form document in an EPR system be stored in the form of XML. From this XML, information in the document needed to produce the UPR can be selected out and converted (from one format to another if necessary), and information to enable display of the document through the UPR can be created.

XML enables "data" to be separated from "format" to be separated from "rendering (display or presentation)." Figure 12 illustrates the three parts of XML: data, format and rendering.

Data. The data part of XML identifies the data making up an automated medical record document with each item of

Data: XML
    <PatientName>Joann Jensen</PatientName>
    <PatientId> 3456789 </PatientId>
    <PatientBirthDate> 1970-07-21 </PatientBirthDate>

Format: XML DTD or XML Schema
    <element name = "PatientBirthDate"
        type = "date">

Rendering: XSL
    On a form, a computer screen, or voice

Figure 12 XML = Data + Format + Rendering.

data enclosed within start and end tags where the tags give the data element a name (e.g., "PatientName" or "PatientId"). Thus the tag allows the piece of data to be identified while the data gives a value (e.g., the "PatientId" has a value of "3456789."

Format. The format part of XML identifies by data element name the data type of the data element. For example the date being of type "date" is stored in the data part in the form YYYY-MM-DD, where YYYY is the year, MM is the numeric month number, and DD is the numeric day number. When there is no corresponding data element name in the format part of the XML, then the data is in terms of characters (e.g., the patient identifier may be a string of, in this case numeric, characters).

Rendering. The rendering part of the XML (XSL) enables XML data to be displayed in a different order than it appears in the data part, in a different format than the format part, and to include or exclude data when the XML data is used for display. Further the XML can use the same data to display different forms of outputs: display in terms of a medical record form, display on a computer screen, or presented as spoken words. For example, for the date stored as "1970-07-21", rendering could be in the form "07/21/1970" and the date can be put on the upper right of a medical record form displayed on a computer screen.

One approach is to have each automated medical record form document use all three parts of XML, in which case the document can be rendered differently than the order of data in the XML data format. An alternative approach is to use the HL7 Clinical Document Architecture standard for clinical documents, CDA, which uses only the data and format parts (Dolin et al. 2001); CDA displays the data in the order it exists in the XML data part formatted according to the XML format part.

Most often XML consists of text but also enables storage of visual and other multimedia information (Westermann and Klas 2003).

3.2.2.2 Partially Standardized Medical Record Documents

In order to partially create the UPR from EPR medical record documents, these EPR medical record documents must collectively have the same data as in the UPR, although they might use different data formats (e.g., medication information in the EPR of a different format than in the UPR, and patient identifiers stored as local medical record numbers in the EPR but universal patient health identifiers in the UPR).

In order to associate EPR medical record documents with a patient, each EPR medical record document must have an identifier of the patient. In order to associate EPR medical record documents with encounters, the document must have information that identifies the encounter. In order to associate an EPR medical record document with a case and/or episode, it must have information to identify the associated case and/or episode. Thus to enable EPR medical record documents to be displayed in the UPR, I propose that all EPR medical records, whether automated forms, scanned forms or diagnostic digital images include information that enables the document to be associated with the patient, with an encounter for an encounter related document, with a case for a case related document, and/or with an episode for an episode related document. Additionally the medical record document type should be given a name (e.g., history and physical) to identify the document type and a locator should be stored in the UPR to locate the document in an EPR system so the document can be retrieved for display in the UPR from the EPR system.

Many EPR medical record documents contain information required by the UPR beyond the *index* information that associates the document with a patient, an encounter, a case or an episode. For example, prescriptions would provide information for UPR medications; and history and physical and progress notes could provide encounter information such as clinicians and diagnoses associated with the encounter. It is proposed that parts of these types of named EPR automated medical record documents (e.g., prescriptions, history and physical, progress notes) have required sets of data agreed-upon by the health care industry while other parts of these types of documents could have data decided by the health care organization. For example, all prescription medical record documents would have the medication and dosage, although the formats of this data in prescription documents in different health care organizations might differ. Such documents with medical industry agreed-upon common data beyond patient, encounter, case or episode index information might include the following types of documents:

- History and physical
- Progress notes
- Physician orders and results (clinical laboratory, pharmacy, anatomic pathology, etc.)
- Prescription and fulfillments of the prescription
- Referral request
- Consultation request
- Referral response
- Consultation response
- Clinician encounter directive to the patient (a proposed new type of document)
- Clinician health problem directive to the patient (a proposed new type of document)
- Some types of case documentation.

The medical industry would agree upon what data elements were required in each of the types of medical record documents. Some data elements may be required to have data while other data elements may optionally have data.

The data supplied in these documents must be sufficient to supply or be converted into UPR information needed. Some data elements may be the same in an EPR document as the data in the UPR and may not require any conversion. Other data, for example, a medication in a prescription document, may have to be converted to the format in the UPR before it is sent to the UPR. A third possibility is that the data could be converted by the UPR rather than in the EPR; the UPR might be given the data in the EPR and told what conversion was required (e.g., a British "Read code" in the

EPR might be sent to the UPR and the UPR, knowing its format, might do a conversion of the Read code into an ICD diagnosis and/or CPT procedure).

Having required data elements in a particular type of EPR medical record and allowing the health care organization to determine the rest of the information allows for a commonality of information in medical documents that enables the UPR to pick up information from the document but still allows health care organizations to customize such documents for their own use.

A partial standardization of medical record documents enables EPR medical record documents to be used to create the UPR and enables these documents to be properly indexed in the UPR (associating the document with a patient, encounter, case or episode).

3.2.2.3 *Types of EPR Medical Records*

Again, there are the following types of medical records in a health care organization (see table 1):

- Automated medical record forms
- Scanned medical record forms
- Diagnostic digital images
- Chart room medical records.

Automated medical record forms. An emerging standard for EPR automated medical record forms (e.g., a history and physical document) is to use XML for the data and formats of the data. Clinical Document Architecture, CDA, is one approach used; data can be displayed sequentially on a form or screen. Adding XSL could produce the data as it looked on a paper form at the health care organization. It is expected that all automated medical record forms would have the information needed to index the document within the UPR and supply the information for the document type within the UPR as well as providing index and data information for the EPR.

Scanned medical record forms. When medical records are scanned, they usually are stored as a picture using TIFF (Wikipedia 2009) format, although other formats are sometimes used such as JPEG or GIF. When such a document is scanned, often the scanning system uses OCR (optical character recognition) software to digitize some of the information on the form (e.g., the patient's medical record number could be at a particular location on the form and read by OCR). In the physical location where the document is scanned, there usually are computer users who look at the scanned form and OCR information and may either correct the OCR information or add additional information from the scanned form. It is expected that this additional or OCR information would include information for EPR and UPR indexes and supply the information for the document type within the UPR.

An emerging standard for communicating an automated or scanned medical record form to other systems for purposes of display is PDF (Portable Document Format) (AIIM 2008). Automated medical record forms thus would be converted from XML to PDF before sending the information for display through the UPR, and scanned medical record forms would be converted from TIFF or other scanned formats to PDF before sending the information for display through the UPR.

Diagnostic digital images. When a machine, such as an x-ray or MRI machine, produces a digital image, the digital image is displayed to a computer user through a computer sys-

Document Type	Typical Storage in EPR	Data Sent to UPR	Proposed Information for Display Through the UPR
Automated form	XML for form (e.g., CDA)	XML with universal data only, converted + name of document + locator for display	PDF converted from XML for form (e.g., CDA)
Scanned form	TIFF scanned image + EPR indexes + EPR data + any added information for UPR indexes + any added information for UPR data	UPR indexes with universal data, converted + UPR data with universal data, converted + name of document + locator for display (possibly sent as XML)	PDF converted from TIFF scanned image
Diagnostic digital image	DICOM image + EPR indexes + EPR data + any added information for UPR indexes + any added information for UPR data	UPR indexes with universal data, converted + UPR data with universal data, converted + name of document + locator for display (possibly sent as XML)	PDF used to transport DICOM image
Chart room document	None (stored in chart room)	An indicator in the encounter that there are chart room medical records	Not displayable

Table 1 Using medical records to create the UPR.

tem. The computer operator can enter additional information to be stored with the digital image. Diagnostic digital images are by standard stored in the form of DICOM (NEMA 2008). PDF can be used to transport DICOM images to outside software systems for display (Colangelo 2009), forming a *wrapper* around the DICOM data. It is expected that all diagnostic digital image documents would have operator added information needed to index the document within the UPR and supply the information for the document type within the UPR.

Chart room documents. Medical records on paper and non-digitized diagnostic images are stored in chart rooms rather than on EPR systems. When a clinician in the health care organization wants to see such documents, he or she makes a request to the chart room to send over the patient's current chart. A clinician in another health care organization may be able to get copies of these paper medical records or diagnostic images upon request.

3.2.2.4 Creation of the UPR Partially from EPR Medical Record Documents

See table 1 again. With sections 3.2.2.1 - 3.2.2.3 providing background information, this section describes how EPR automated, scanned and diagnostic image medical record documents can be used to create the basic information in the UPR and to enable the UPR to display these documents.

Indexes are data that can be associated with a document to allow it to be retrieved. For example, to retrieve all documents for a patient, each document must be associated with a patient identifier. To retrieve all documents for a patient and encounter, each document must be associated with a patient identifier and encounter identifiers, perhaps, patient identifier, start date, start time and medical facility locator. The EPR must associate indexes with its documents to store and retrieve them within the EPR system, and the UPR must create indexes to store and retrieve information within the UPR. In the UPR there could be indexes for cases and episodes.

An automated medical record form is assumed to be initially stored in the EPR within XML, with the ability to convert it to PDF format for display in the UPR. The EPR

XML would include the document type, all the information required for EPR and UPR indexing, and UPR data required by the document type (e.g., prescription, progress note) and other EPR data. Before sending the XML information to the UPR, also probably in XML format, EPR data not required by the UPR would be stripped out, and data for the UPR would be converted to universal data formats if necessary. Included with the XML data sent to the UPR would be a locator of the PDF document in the EPR (or alternatively, a locator of the EPR XML document that could be converted to PDF)—the locator would allow the UPR to later request the PDF document for display through the UPR.

A scanned medical record form is assumed to be initially stored in the EPR in TIFF format with the TIFF format document being able to be converted to PDF format. When the document is scanned, OCR could strip out data from the scanned document to be stored with the document, and the computer user viewing the document after it was scanned can type in additional information or correct the OCR data. This additional information would include document type, EPR and UPR indexes, additional data used by the EPR, and any additional data for the UPR. The document type, UPR indexes, data to be used by UPR, and a locator of the TIFF PDF document in the EPR (or alternatively, the locator of the TIFF document that could be converted to PDF) would be sent to the UPR—the locator would allow the UPR to later request the PDF document for display through the UPR.

A diagnostic digital image is stored in the EPR in DICOM format, with DICOM being the national standard for digitized diagnostic images. When the diagnostic image is created (e.g., x-ray or MRI), it is sent to a computer system. The computer system can add information to be stored with the diagnostic image. Like for a scanned document, this additional data could include document type, EPR and UPR indexes, additional data used by the EPR, and any additional data for the UPR. The document type, UPR indexes, data to be used by UPR, and a locator of the DICOM document in the EPR would be sent to the UPR. Upon request of the UPR, the DICOM image would be put in a PDF *wrapper* to be transported over the secure health care network for display through the UPR.

Chart room documents would not be displayable through the UPR. When there are chart room documents to be created during the encounter, the encounter information sent to the UPR at the beginning of an encounter could contain an indicator that chart room documents exist for the encounter but not identify them.

3.2.3 Changes to an EPR System to Support the UPR

Incorporating a particular brand of EPR system with the UPR through the secure health care network would require changes to the EPR system, including the following:

- **A secure health care network:** The EPR system should communicate with the UPR(s) through a secure health care network.

- **Universal patient health number assignment and look up:** The EPR should be able to look up, verify and request assignment of a universal patient health number to a patient by communications with an "assigning authority," a service at a national or international level through the secure health care network to assign or look up a universal patient health number. (Assignment of an individual with a universal patient health number prior to any visits, and perhaps including it on a smart card carried by the individual or recording it together with patient biometrics (e.g., palm prints) would decrease the chances of any errors in assignment or misidentification of the patient.)

- **The UPR information for a patient can be displayed for a clinician caring for the patient:** Through the secure health care network the UPR information for a patient identified by a universal patient health number can be displayed, and automated, scanned, and diagnostic digital image medical records for a selected encounter can be retrieved for display.

- **The EPR sends encounter information to the UPR before sending any encounter medical records:** Through the secure health care network, the EPR could send encounter information to the UPR during an encounter. Together with the encounter information, the EPR could identify that there are chart room (off-line) medical records that will be associated with the encounter. Encounter software systems interfaced with the EPR could send encounter information to the EPR that sends it to the UPR. The clinician can associate the current encounter with a case or episode of care.

- **The EPR sends medical record information to the UPR to enable updating of the UPR and later display of the medical records:** For each automated form, scanned form, diagnostic digital image medical record created during an encounter, the corresponding information in column 3 of table 1 will be sent by the EPR to the UPR through the secure health care network. This information will update the

UPR and enable display of the medical records through the UPR upon retrieval from the EPR.

- **The UPR can be redisplayed for verification after an encounter:** After an encounter through the secure health care network, the UPR information can be redisplayed, enabling the clinician to verify that the encounter information was correctly recorded in the UPR. At any time during an encounter, the clinician should be able to indicate that the encounter is part of an existing case or episode; at the end of the encounter, the EPR system should query the UPR to see if there are existing cases or episodes and, if there is, give the clinician a choice of associating the encounter with the case or episode.

- **The UPR can be updated by the clinician:** The clinician can make changes to the UPR (e.g., significant health problems, current medications, etc.) as agreed upon by the medical community and designers of the UPR system.

- **An EPR could send and receive referral and consultation requests and send referral and consultation responses through the UPR:** Referral and consultation requests and responses for clinicians could be sent and received through the UPR. A large health care organization may wish to only use this send and receive capability for referrals and consultations using the UPR secure health care network when the referrals and consultations are for outside health care organizations.

- **Creation of a new case or episode, or retirement of an old case:** The EPR should be modified to be able to request the UPR to start a new case or start a new episode after verifying that an existing open case and/or episode does not exist. The EPR should be modified to enable an authorized clinician to retire a case indicating that it is no longer applicable for care of the patient.

- **The EPR should be modified to enable creation of a care plan or outcome to associate with a case or episode in the UPR:** After the clinician creates a case, selects a case from the UPR, creates an episode or selects an episode, an authorized clinician can create and associate a care plan or outcome medical document through the EPR to be included in the UPR. Included with an episode care plan would also be indications for a patient to have such a treatment, goals of the episode, risks of treatment, and the prognosis for the patient after the episode; this information should be provided to the patient at the start of an episode.

- **The EPR should be modified to enable a clinician to close an episode of care identifying the final outcome of the episode:** When care is completed for an episode of care, the clinician through the EPR system can tell the UPR to close the episode; together with this closure would be a recording of the final outcome of the episode. As a quality control check and part of his or her duty of monitoring a case and associated episodes, a primary care physician can later add his or her analysis of the outcome of the episode of care within the case or, if no case, within the episode.

- **Allergy alert:** Upon EPR request of the UPR (usually at the start of an encounter), the UPR should send back any patient allergies.

- **Medication interactions:** Upon EPR request of the UPR with the EPR identification of a medication that would be ordered (usually just after the clinician enters the medication and dosage), the UPR should send back to the EPR, and the clinician through the EPR, an indication of any drug interaction of the current medication with past medications or of any drug allergy related to the current medication.

- **Duplicate orders:** Upon EPR request of the UPR with the EPR identification of an order (e.g., clinical laboratory test, medication), the UPR should identify that the order might be a possible duplicate order. This EPR request would be most often made after the initiation of an order by the clinician but before it is completed.

- **EPR display of UPR information for the patient, allowing entrance of patient responses to care:** An EPR system should be changed to display UPR information of interest to the patient, and allow a patient to enter a response to information for a recent encounter, including allowing a patient to amend medical records. This capability would be provided either through the Internet or a health care organization Intranet connected to an EPR system. Depending upon agreements of the medical community and designers of the UPR, the patient may be able to selectively update some types of UPR information.

- **Adverse events:** A patient and a clinician who cared for a patient should be able to record an adverse event through the EPR to be sent to the UPR, to record the adverse event through the Internet directly to the UPR, optionally associating the adverse event with a past encounter. Adverse events could include adverse reactions to vaccinations or medications, procedures that caused harm, nosocomial infections (infections that occurred in a hospital), or injuries caused by a consumer product. To whom adverse events would be reported should be determined by the government together with industry and medical organizations.

- **UPR presentation options:** The UPR can be presented in two forms: for the clinician caring for the patient and for the patient. Additionally, the UPR can either present and receive updated information through the Internet or can communicate with an EPR system for the EPR system to display UPR information for the clinician or patient and to send back updated UPR information from the clinician or patient.

4

CONCLUSIONS

In an article in the *New England Journal of Medicine*
(Porter 2009), Michael E. Porter, Ph.D. states that health
care reform will not be successful unless "the central focus
[of medical care] is increasing value for patients—the health
outcomes achieved per dollar spent." He argues that some
of the ways to do this are:

- **Measure outcomes and reimburse using out-comes adjusted for the patient's medical condi-tion:** "Measure outcomes of care in a sophisticated way, basing payment on outcomes. Outcomes must be measured over the full cycle of care for a medical condition, not separately for each intervention. Outcomes must be adjusted for patients' initial con-ditions to eliminate bias against patients with com-plex cases."

- **Prevention and wellness:** "Invest in the delivery of prevention, wellness, screening, and routine health maintenance services as the current health care system under invests in these services relative to their value."

- **Medical condition management and team-based care:** "Reorganize care delivery around med-ical conditions, with care delivery using integrated practice units that encompass all the skills and ser-vices required over the full cycle of care for a medi-cal condition. For chronic conditions, bundled payments should cover extended periods of care and include responsibility for evaluating and addressing complications."

- **Eliminate redundancy:** "Eliminate hyperfragmentation and duplication of services."

- **Make better use of physicians who specialize in less common medical conditions:** "In order to achieve high value, providers need a sufficient volume of cases of a given medical condition to allow for the development of deep expertise, integrated teams, and tailored facilities. In particular this applies to rare medical conditions. Achieving this volume may require care to be provided over larger geographic areas than currently."

- **Support cases, standards of care, and continuity-of-care:** "To achieve value improvement, electronic medical record systems need to support integrated care and outcome measurement and to provide an architecture for aggregating data for each patient over time and across providers, and protocols for seamless communication among systems."

- **Support and improve health care industry standards:** "Finalize and then continuously update health information technology (HIT) standards that include precise data definitions (for diagnoses and treatments, for example)."

- **Independent organizations to define and enforce standards:** "Some new organizations (or combinations of existing ones) will be needed: a new independent body to oversee outcome measurement and reporting, a single entity to review and set HIT standards, and possibly a third body to establish rules for bundled reimbursement. Medicare may be able to take the lead in some areas; for example, Medicare could require experience reporting by providers or combine Parts A and B into one payment."

- **Patient involvement in care:** "Consumers must become much more involved in their health and health care."

The universal patient medical record (UPR) supports all these objectives. However, for the UPR to do so, clinicians must change the way they provide care, patients must be more involved in care and agencies should provide guidance in identifying standards of care and best practices for the clinicians to follow. Changes in health care with a UPR would include the following:

- **Clinician use of an EPR:** Electronic patient record systems (EPRs) must first be widely used by health care organizations before a UPR can be implemented.

- **Clinician use of the UPR:** During an encounter, a clinician should review the UPR information with the patient and make any corrections. At the end of the encounter, the clinician should verify that encounter information was correctly recorded.

- **Clinician directives for the patient:** After an encounter, the clinician should create an encounter directive for the patient in the language a patient can understand. The encounter directive could be printed and given to the patient after the encounter, or the patient could later view the encounter directive through the Internet or an Intranet. The clinician could also create a health problem directive for the patient related to one of the patient's significant health problems for patient review. The physician should also be able to report on adverse events such as adverse reactions to vaccinations or medications or nosocomial infections (infections that occurred while in the hospital).

- **Patient information and patient response to care:** The patient should be able to review their medical records and information in the UPR (through the EPR via the Internet or Intranet). After an encounter, the patient should be able amend their medical records and respond to care—in particular, the patient can challenge that the care stated was the care given. The patient may be selectively able to update UPR information. Through the UPR, the patient would be able to report on adverse events such as adverse reactions to vaccinations or medications or nosocomial infections or injury-causing consumer products.

- **Case management for chronic and long-term conditions:** For care for a chronic or other condition over time, a clinician should open a case and create an overall care plan for the condition. All later clinicians should follow the care plan. When there are multiple chronic conditions, a clinician responsible for the care plan for one medical condition should consult with the clinician(s) responsible for the care plans for the other medical conditions to address co-morbidities within each care plan. Within the case, other clinicians should be able to record second opinions.

- **Episode management for periods of intense care:** For an intense period of care for a medical condition, a clinician should open an episode and create an episode care plan consistent with any case care plan. Included with the episode care plan would be indications for a patient to have the treatment, goals of the episode, risks of treatment, and the prognosis for the patient after the episode; this information should be provided to the patient prior to the episode. The acuity of the patient could be included in the episode to identify patients that are more difficult to treat. At the end of the episode, the clinician should close the episode and add the final outcome of the episode. After an episode of care was performed by a specialty provider, a primary care provider can add an independent outcome of the episode to a case or the episode. Excluding the identity of the patient, successful episode care plans should be able to be shared with other health care organizations.

- **Periodic recording of outcomes:** Case outcomes should be recorded during periodic visits, in particular to check for critical points in the progression of a medical condition. This may apply to episodes also.

- **Government and health care organization support of standards of care and best practices:** The government, medical associations together with health care organizations should produce standards of care that could be used in case and episode care plans. The US government and medical associations should evaluate standards of care to determine best practices based upon evidence and provide a data base of standards of care and care plans. New standards of care should be evaluated using clinical trials. As diagnoses (or diagnoses together with biomarkers) become finer, additional standards of care should be created.

- **Process improvements to avoid medical errors:** Methods for avoiding medical errors should be identified by the industry and included in episode care plans (e.g., Atul Gawande's surgery checklist (Gawande 2009)). In order to exchange ideas of best practices and processes to avoid medical errors, health care organizations may want to view each other's episode care plans with identification of the patient excluded.

- **Pharmacists more involved in patient care:** The UPR could provide information to support patient-pharmacist consultations: it could provide a medical history of the patient including current medications. When a patient is taking multiple medications, it can allow the pharmacist, possibly with the consultation of physicians, to develop a medication administration schedule for the patient.

- **Possible interactive team care:** The UPR for a patient could potentially be available to two clinicians collaborating in care of a patient.

- **Display of disease progression and biomarkers over time:** Clinicians will be able to record and display biomarkers over time (e.g., PSA) including a series of diagnostic images over time for a body area to identify disease progression (e.g., the left knee). This information can be used to chart the progress of a disease and to identify critical points in the progression of the disease.

REFERENCES

Adams, Jonathan. 2009. Healthcare, a Global Survey: In Taiwan, your medical file on a card. *The Christian Science Monitor*, October 10, 2009.

AHRQ. *Prevention and management of hip fracture in older people. A national clinical guideline.* FirstGov 2006 [cited. Available from www.guideline.gov.

AIIM. *The Enterprise Content Management Association. PDF Healthcare Overview: A Guide to Safe Access and Transport of Health Information.* 2008 [cited. Available from http://www.aiim.org/documents/standards/pdfhealthcareoverview.pdf.

ASTM. 2009. *ASTM Book of Standards Volume 24.01 Health Care Informatics.* Edited by A. International, *ASTM Book of Standards.* West Conshohocken, PA: ASTM (American Society for Testing and Materials).

Bohannon, John. 2009. The Theory? Diet Causes Violence. The Lab. Prison. *Science*, 25 September 2009, 1614-1616.

BSCS. 2007. *Glossary.* BSCS 2003 [cited September 27, 2007 2007]. Available from http://science.education.nih.gov/supplements/nih3/alcohol/other/glossary.htm.

Burton, Robert. 2008. *On Being Certain—Believing You Are Right Even When You're Not.* New York: St. Martin's Press.

Campeau, Deb. 2007. Establishing an Effective Workplace Wellness Program: A Strategic Opportunity. In *McLaughlin & Smoak INFORUM*: Trident Health System.

Canadian Institutes of Health Research. *The Brain from Top to Bottom* 2002 [cited. Available from http://thebrain.mcgill.ca/flash/index_a.html.

Carlsen, E., A. Gwercman, N. Keiding, and N. Skakkebaek. 1992. Evidence for decreasing quality of semen during past 50 years. *British Medical Journal* 305 (6854):6854-6858.

Colangelo, John. *PDF in Healthcare: Personal Health Records and DICOM Images—The Future is Now* 2009 [cited September 16, 2009. Available from http://www.eradimaging.com/site/article.cfm?ID=328.

Colavita, Francis. 2006. *Sensation, Perception, and the Aging Process*: The Teaching Company.

Dolin, Robert, Liora Alschuler, Calvin Beebe, Paul Biron, Sandra Boyer, Daniel Essin, Elliot Kimber, Tom Lincoln, and John Mattison. 2001. The HL7 Clinical Document Architecture. *Journal of the American Medical Informatics Association* 8 (552-569).

Esserman, Laura, Yiwey Shieh, and Ian Thompson. 2009. Rethinking Screening for Breast Cancer and Prostate Cancer. *JAMA* 302 (15):1685-1692.

Farmer, Richard, and Ross Lawrenson. 2004. *Lecture Notes on Epidemiology and Public Health*. 5Rev Ed ed. Malden, Oxford: Blackwell Science Ltd.

Gawande, A. (2009). *The Checklist Manifesto: How to Get Things Right*, Metropolitan Books.

Kim, J., B. Greber, M. Arauzo-Bravo, J. Meyer, K. Park, H. Zaehres, and H. Scholer. 2009. Direct reprogramming of human neural stem cells. *Nature* (October 4).

Lawrence, David. 2003. *From Chaos to Care: The Promise of Team-Based Medicine*. Reprint edition ed. Cambridge, MA: Da Capo Press.

Magrinos, Ana, Jose Verdugo, and Bruce McEwen. 1997. Chronic stress alters synaptic terminal structure in hippocampus. *Proceedings of the National Academy of Sciences* 94 (25):7.

Mahar, Maggie. 2006. *Money-Driven Medicine: The Real Reason Health Care Costs So Much*: Harper Collins.

McCallum, J. 1993. What is an outcome and why look at them? *Critical Public Health* 4 (4):1.

McGuire, Michael. 2004. *Steps Toward a Universal Patient Medical Record: A Project Plan to Develop One*: Universal Publishers.

———. 2006. Incorporating an EPR system with a Universal Patient Record. *Journal of Medical Systems* 30 (4):9.

Microsoft ® Encarta ® 2007. © 1993-2007 Microsoft Corporation.

Mitchell, Susan, Joan Teno, Dan Kiely, Michele Shaffer, Richard Jones, Holly Prigerson, Ladislav Volicer, Jane Givens, and Mary Hamel. 2009. The Clinical Course of Advanced Dementia. *New England Journal of Medicine* 361:1529-1538.

NEMA. *DICOM, Digital Imaging and Communications for Medicine* 2008 [cited. Available from http://medical.nema.org/.

NIH. 2000. Summary of Biomarkers Knowledge System Meeting—September 8, 2000: National Institutes of Health.

Norden, Jeanette. 2007. *Understanding the Brain*. Chantilly, Virginia: The Great Courses.

Oasis. *Health Level Seven Releases Updated Clinical Document Architecture (CDA) Specification.* 2004 [cited November 4, 2009. Available from http://xml.coverpages.org/ni2004-08-20-a.html.

Pelengaris, Steller, and Mike Khan. 2006. Introduction. In *The Molecular Biology of Cancer*, edited by S. Pelengaris and M. Khan. Malden, MA: Blackwell Publishing.

Porter, Michael. 2009. A Strategy for Health Care Reform—Toward a Value-Based System. *New England Journal of Medicine* 361 (2):4.

Ramiya, V. K., M. Maraist, K. E. Arfors, D. A. Schatz, A. B. Peck, and J. G. Cornelius. 2000. Reversal of insulin-dependent diabetes using islets generated in vitro from pancreatic stem cells. *Nat. Med.* 6 (3):5.

Russell, Louise. 1986. *Is Prevention Better Than Cure?, Studies in Social Economics*. Washington, D.C.: Brookings Institution Press.

Sackett, David L., R. Brian Haynes, Peter Tugwell, and Gordon H. Guyatt. 1991. *Clinical Epidemiology: A Basic Science for Clinical Medicine*. 2nd Bk&Acc edition ed. Philadelphia, PA: Lippincott Williams & Wilkins.

Sell, Steward. 1990. Is There a Liver Stem Cell? *Cancer Research* 50:5.

Smith, Stephanie. 2009. *Doctors grow organs from patients' own cells* (April 5, 2006). Cable News Network (CNN) 2006 [cited 2009]. Available from http://www.cnn.com/2006/HEALTH/conditions/04/03/engineered.organs/index.html.

Starfield, Barbara. 2000. Medical Errors—A Leading Cause of Death. *Journal of the American Medical Association (JAMA)* 284 (4).

Stein, Rob. 2004. Study confirms that stress helps speed aging. *washingtonpost.com*, November 30, 2004.

Taubes, Gary. 2009. Prosperity's Plague. *Science*, 17 July 2009, 5.

Thorn, Caroline, Teri Klein, and Russ Altman. 2009. Codeine and morphine pathway. *Pharmacogenetics and Genomics* 19 (7):556-558.

Timmermans, S., and A. Mauck. 2005. The promises and pitfalls of evidence-based medicine. *Health Aff (Millwood)* 24 (1):18-28.

University of Southern California. *USC/Norris Comprehensive Cancer Center Glossary* 2009 [cited November 1, 2009. Available from http://ccnt.hsc.usc.edu/glossary/.

University of Wisconsin-Madison. (2003). "HIPAA Privacy Rule Research Guidance." 2009, from http://hipaa.wisc.edu/ResearchGuide/index.html.

US Department of Health and Human Services. 2006. Alzheimer's Disease Genetics Fact Sheet, edited by N. I. o. Aging: National Institutes of Health.

Wade, Nicolas. 2006. Stem Cells May Be Key to Cancer. *New York Times*, February 21, 2006.

Watters, Ethan. 2006. DNA is not destiny: Forget everything you knew about genes, disease and heredity. The new science of epigenetics shows why your genetic code does not determine your fate. *DISCOVER-NEW YORK-* 27 (11):32-37.

Wikipedia. 2009. *Acute Care 2009* [cited November 4, 2009]. Available from http://en.wikipedia.org/wiki/Acute_care

————. *Digital Imaging and Communications in Medicine* 2009 [cited November 4, 2009. Available from http://en.wikipe-dia.org/wiki/Digital_Imaging_and_Communications_in_Medicine.

————. *Epigenetics* 2009 [cited. Available from http://en.wikipedia.org/wiki/Epigenetic.

————. *Graphics Interchange Format* 2009 [cited November 6, 2009. Available from http://en.wikipedia.org/wiki/Graphics_Interchange_Format.

————. *JPEG* 2009 [cited. Available from http://en.wikipedia.org/wiki/JPEG.

————. *Knee replacement* 2009 [cited 2009]. Available from http://en.wikipedia.org/wiki/Knee_replacement.

————. *Pharmacogenetics* 2009 [cited 2009]. Available from http://en.wikipedia.org/wiki/Pharmacogenetics.

————. *Prion* 2009 [cited 2009] Available from http://en.wikipedia.org/wiki/Prion.

————. *Tagged Image File Format* 2009 [cited 2009]. Available from http://en.wikipedia.org/wiki/Tagged_Image_File_Format.

GLOSSARY

acuity: The intensity of nursing care required to meet the needs of a patient; a higher acuity indicates the need for longer and more frequent nurse visits and more supplies and equipment. Acuity in this book is also applied to evaluating the intensity of care that needs to be given by a physician or other healthcare practitioners during an episode of care; this acuity measurement could be used to structure payments for care so that healthcare practitioners are not disadvantaged monetarily in taking more difficult to treat patients.

acute care: "Treatment of a disease for only a short period of time in which a patient is treated for a brief but severe episode of illness." (Wikipedia 2009)

admission: The formal acceptance by a hospital of a patient who is to be provided room, board, and continuous nursing services in an area of the hospital where patients generally stay at least overnight.

adult stem cell: Stem cells found in the human body that can only turn into certain specialized types of cells rather than all types of human cells. Also called "somatic stem cells."

advance directive: Written instructions a patient has prepared for medical personnel to inform them of the patient's wishes for treatments and care when the patient is incapacitated, especially regarding life-sustaining treatment if the patient's condition becomes irreversible. An advance directive is a legal document prepared when the individual is competent and able to make decisions. Advance directives only apply when the patient is incapacitated and enable to make decisions for herself or himself.

ADT (admission, discharge and transfer) system: A clinical system for recording admissions to a hospital, discharges from a hospital and transfers within a hospital and for maintaining the hospital census.

Agency for Healthcare Research (AHRQ): An agency of the United States government that is part of the U.S. Department of Health & Human Services whose mission is to improve the quality, safety, efficiency, and effectiveness of health care for all Americans. AHCPR has developed clinical practice guidelines based upon "evidence-based medicine."

allergy: A concerning reaction of the immune system to a substance.

amino acid: A building block for a polypeptide, and one of the building blocks for a subsequently formed protein.

angiogenesis: Fast growing cells such as cancer cells sending out signals to form new blood vessels. One approach to fighting cancer is to stop growth of these blood vessels.

assigning authority: An entity who has the power to assign a universal patient health identifier to a patient or to give information that verifies that a given individual is the one assigned that identifier.

automated medical record form: A medical record form created from clinical information entered through an EPR system.

best practice: A standard-of-care that is believed to be more effective at delivering a particular outcome for a particular medical condition than any other standard-of-care.

bind: To form a chemical bond.

biomarker: "Cellular, biochemical, molecular, or genetic characteristics or alterations by which a normal, abnormal, or simply biologic process can be recognized, or monitored."(NIH 2000)

biometrics: Identifying a person based up measurable biological characteristics such as voice, fingerprints, palm print, signature, etc.

capitation: A method of payment for health services in which a health care provider is paid a fixed amount for each person served over a given time period regardless of the actual services provided.

care plan: A document identifying the tasks and responsibilities of all those involved in caring for a person over a significant period of time for a particular medical condition for medical purposes.

case: "An organized (automated or non-automated) system for managing the delivery of health care to an individual for a medical condition or conditions that includes assessment and development of a plan of care, coordination of services, referrals and follow-ups."(McGuire 2004)

cell: "The smallest structure capable of basic life processes. All living things are composed of cells." (Microsoft ® Encarta ® 2007)

cell nucleus: A membrane-bound structure in the cells of humans that contains the genetic information including chromosomes and DNA embedded in the chromosomes.

cell signaling: The sending of a hormone or other molecules from one cell to other cells where receptors in the other cells bind with the hormone or molecules, thus receiving the signal.

cell wall (membrane): The outer layer surrounding a human cell that protects the cell from its surrounding environment. The cell wall may embed receptors.

chart room: A physical location for the storage of paper medical records or non-digitized diagnostic images such as x-rays.

chart room medical record: A paper medical record or non-digitized diagnostic image such as an x-ray or MRI.

chronic condition: A medical condition that lasts or keeps coming back over a long period of time.

(HL7) Clinical Document Architecture (CDA): "An XML-based document markup standard that specifies the structure and semantics of clinical documents for the purpose of exchange." (Oasis 2004)

clinical pathway: "A structured way to identify care activities and caregiver work flow needed to care for a patient with a particular condition or disease. Paths through a clinical pathway can be adjusted for the particular needs of an individual patient." (McGuire 2004)

clinical summary: "A summary of clinical information about a patient, which may include demographics information, significant health problems, past encounters, primary care physicians and other significant caregivers, and medications." (McGuire 2004)

clinical trial: A formal method used to determine if a diagnostic, treatment or prevention measure is safe, effective, and better than a current standard-of-care.

comparative effectiveness: The direct comparison of existing health care interventions to determine which work best for which patients and which pose the greatest benefits and least harm.

co-morbidities: The presence of one or more medical conditions in addition to a given medical condition.

consultation: Process in which the help of a specialist is sought to provide advice or care for a patient. A request for a consultation is often accompanied by a referral; see "referral."

continuity-of-care: The coordination of care received by a patient over time where care could be given by one or many different healthcare practitioners.

critical point: "A time before which therapy is more effective or easier to apply than afterwards." (Sackett et al. 1991)

cytoplasm: The contents of a cell excluding its nucleus.

de-identified information: A HIPAA term to identify health information from which protected health information has been removed, removing data that could be used to identify a patient.

dendrite: A branched extension of a nerve cell neuron that receives neurotransmitter chemicals from dendrites in other neurons and conducts these signals to the cell body.

diagnostic digital image: A diagnostic image in numerical form so it can be stored and used in a computer.

diagnostic image: A picture from an x-ray, MRI or other medical device used for diagnosis.

DICOM (Digital Imaging and Communications for Medicine): "A standard for handling, storing, printing, and transmitting medical image information." (Wikipedia 2009)

differentiation: "Parts of genetic information in cells selectively being turned on or off depending upon the individual cell's role in the whole organism." (Microsoft ® Encarta ® 2007)

discharge: Termination of a period of inpatient hospitalization through the formal release of the inpatient by the hospital or the release of a patient from the emergency department.

disease progression map: "A diagram to identify the progression of a disease over time and current status of the patient in the disease progression, identifying critical points in the progression of the disease." (McGuire 2004) A disease progression map may be used in combination with a case or a care plan.

distributed: Describing a computer system that consists of multiple autonomous computers that communicate through a computer network.

DNA (deoxyribonucleic acid): "The genetic material of all cellular organisms and most viruses." (Microsoft ® Encarta ® 2007)

DNA methylation: The addition of a methyl group to a stretch of DNA, which can lock, or silence, that gene. If methylation silences a gene that normally would control cell growth or prompt the cell to commit suicide, then the cell could grow unchecked—the hallmark of cancer (University of Southern California 2009).

electronic patient record system (EPR): A system to automate and replace the paper patient medical record with entrance of information by clinicians caring for the patient. Such an EPR system often has interfaces with other clinical and encounter software systems such as clinical laboratory and hospital admission systems to receive orders and send back order results and to identify new encounters.

embryonic stem cells (ESC): A type of stem cell that occurs in embryos that has the potential to divide to produce all other types of human cells.

encounter: "A face-to-face interaction between a patient and a healthcare provider. In some cases this may also include an interaction via a phone call or television if this takes the place of the face-to-face interaction. Encounters could include all of the following: an inpatient stay, outpatient visit, emergency department visit, advice nurse call, a phone call between a patient and a physician, a home health visit, a skilled nursing facility (SNF) visit." (McGuire 2004)

epidemic: Occurring suddenly in numbers clearly in excess of normal expectancy; said especially of infectious diseases but applied also to any disease, injury, or other health-related event occurring in such outbreaks.

epidemiology: Study of the occurrence, distribution, and causes of disease and the application of this study to the control of health problems.

epigenetics: "Refers to changes in phenotype (appearance) or gene expression caused by mechanisms other than changes in the underlying DNA sequence." (Wikipedia 2009) By contrast, see "mutation."

episode (of care): A time period of intense care for a medical condition. Whereas there may be a case for a medical condition over a long period of time (e.g., a knee injury), there may be times where there is a period of intense care (e.g., a surgery on the knee). The episode would have its own case structure with its own care plan and outcomes.

evidence-based medicine: The practice of medicine that aims to apply "the best available evidence gained from the scientific method to medical decision making." (Timmermans and Mauck 2005)

(gene) expression: The production of an RNA or protein from a gene that results from gene transcription, the combining of amino acids to form a polypeptide and/or the folding of polypeptides and possible combination with other molecules.

(protein) expression: Gene expression that produces a protein.

gene therapy: "Manipulating genes in cells—often using viruses—in order to produce proteins that change the functions of a cell." (Microsoft ® Encarta ® 2007)

genome: The blueprint for the creation of proteins or RNAs within the interior of the cell.

Graphics Interchange Format (GIF): "A bitmap image format that was introduced by CompuServe in 1987 and has since come into widespread usage on the World Wide Web due to its wide support and portability." (Wikipedia 2009)

gold standard: The intervention generally believed to be the best available option.

HIPAA (The Health Insurance Portability and Accountability Act of 1996 for Medicare and Medicaid programs): A federal bill that includes standards for security and electronic signatures, provider identifiers and taxonomy, electronic transfers, and employer identifiers.

histone: A protein structure involved in the coiling chromosomes (where a chromosome is a rod like structure in the cell nucleus containing DNA, where the chromosomes constitute the genome).

history and physical (H&P): Documentation of health history and physical examination. The purpose of the health history is to collect "subjective" data, what the person says about himself or herself. The physical examination collects "objective" data, a record of the clinician's examination of the patient and of diagnostic measurements.

HL7 (Health Level 7): Messaging standards for information exchange between disparate clinical, administrative and financial computer systems for the healthcare industry, developed by ANSI. "7" refers to the seventh level of the OSI/ISO interconnection reference model. HL7 is also the group who created the Clinical Document Architecture; see "Clinical Document Architecture."

HMO (Health Maintenance Organization): A corporate entity (profit or non-profit) that provides comprehensive health care for members for a fixed periodic payment specified in advance. See "capitation."

hormone: A chemical created by one of a human body's cells that allows communication with other cells.

hospice care: The same as "palliative care."

index: An object consisting of identified data elements in a relational database table that is used to control the order in which the table is accessed or stored; a way to order documents so they can be presented back in a logical order, such as by date, last then first name, etc.

induced pluripotent stem cell (iPSC): ESC-like stem cells created by changing the genes of adult stem cells resulting in cells that are pluripotent. See "pluripotent."

inpatient: Patient admitted for treatment within a hospital over the course of more than one day.

Internet: Worldwide network of interconnected computers. Uses the TCP/IP communications protocol.

intervention: An action that produces an effect or that is intended to alter the course of a disease process.

Intranet: A private computer network based upon the data communication standards of the public Internet.

JPEG: "A commonly used method of compression for photographic images." (Wikipedia 2009)

(gene) knock down: Techniques by which the expression of one or more of an organism's genes is reduced, such as use of RNAi.

life care path: "A clinical pathway identifying preventive care for an individual over a long period of time." (McGuire 2004)

managed care: An arrangement where a third-party payer (such as an insurance company, federal government, or corporation) mediates between physicians and patients, negotiating fees for service and overseeing the types of care given.

(patient) medical record: A written or automated transcription of information obtained from a patient, guardian or medical professional concerning a patient's health history, diagnostic tests, diagnoses, treatment and prognosis. Also the total of such information for a given individual—a longitudinal patient medical record.

molecular medicine: See "personalized medicine."

mutation: A change in the DNA base sequence in a cell.

MRI (Magnetic Resonance Imaging): A medical imaging technique that uses magnetic forces to obtain detailed images of the body that does not require radiation.

neuron: Cells that are "responsible for the transmission and analysis of all electrochemical communication within the brain and other parts of the nervous system." (Microsoft ® Encarta ® 2007)

neurotransmitter: A chemical that enables communication between neurons.

nosocomial infection: An infection acquired in a hospital.

optical character recognition (OCR): A process wherein a printed page is scanned and the resulting image of the page or line is interpreted and translated into a sequence of characters that can be used within a computer program.

(medical) order: A request for service from a clinician to an ancillary department for a particular patient, which may be hand delivered to a performing area or may be sent from a clinical application where the order was created to another clinical application where the performing area is located.

outcome: A measurement of the value of a particular course of therapy.

outpatient: A patient seen in a health care organization not seen as an inpatient.

palliative care: Treatment, usually provided at the end of a patient's life, to relieve the symptoms of a disease to make the patient more comfortable rather than to provide a cure. Palliative care is provided in an end-of-life situation where the comfort of the patient is of more concern that providing "heroic" treatments that might extend the life of the patient for a short time at the expense of causing the patient greater misery.

partially standardized medical record documents: A suggestion of this book to have certain commonly used EPR medical record document types (e.g., H&P) all have the provision for certain types of data needed by the UPR (e.g., diagnoses and clinicians for an H&P). The data need not be in the format required by the UPR but must be convertible to that needed in the UPR. The data may or may not be required. Other parts of the document type can have any additional data required by the health care organization; thus the EPR medical record document is only "partially standardized."

pandemic: An epidemic over a wide geographic area.

past medical history: Any encounters or illnesses the patient has had in the past along with the treatments administered or operations performed.

patient: One who is sick with, or being treated for, an illness or injury.

personal health record: A patient-maintained past medical history available on-line on the Internet.

personalized medicine: Use of the genetic information of an individual or of the inter-workings of that individual's cells to determine how to best provide patient care, thus providing care tailored for that patient.

pharmacogenetics: "The study of genetic variation that gives rise to differing responses to drugs." (Wikipedia 2009)

physician: Health care professional who has the degree of Doctor of Medicine (MD) or Doctor of Osteopath (OD) and is licensed to provide medical, surgical and other treatment.

pluripotent: The ability of a stem cell to produce any type of cell within the human body except for those related to some embryonic tissues such as the placenta.

polypeptide: A chain of linked amino acids that can fold and combine with other molecules to form proteins.

preliminary design: A preliminary design is a first draft of how to construct a software and hardware system. Its principal uses are to verify that requirements for the system as determined by the users of the system have been satisfied, and to serve as a framework and initial specifications for the final design. (Note that the concept of developing a "preliminary design" for a to-be-developed software system was introduced by the United States Air Force.)

prescription: Authorized order for medication, therapy, or a therapeutic device. It is signed by a physician or other practitioner licensed by law to prescribe such a drug, therapy or device.

preventive care: Interventions directed toward preventing illness and promoting health.

primary care: The first contact in a given episode of illness that leads to a decision regarding a course of action to resolve the health problem.

primary care physician: A physician responsible for overseeing and coordinating all aspects of a patient's care. A primary care physician is usually a family practitioner, general internist, pediatrician and sometimes an OB/GYN. The PCP in an HMO initiates most referrals for specialty care.

prion: "An infectious agent that is composed primarily of protein. To date, all such agents that have been discovered propagate by transmitting a misfolded protein state." (Wikipedia 2009)

progress notes: A document recording notes of the patient's progress. An initial medical examination is recorded in a History and Physical; subsequent encounters result in recording the patient's progress in progress notes.

protected health information (PHI): A term used by HIPAA to mean any health information that directly or indirectly identifies a patient (e.g., this woman had octuplets).

protein: A folded macromolecule composed of one or more polypeptides and possibly other molecules.

public health: Community efforts to improve the health of the community through health education, the detection and prevention of disease, and the control of communicable diseases.

Read Classification System (RCS) or Read Code: A coding system used in the United Kingdom that is a superset of several international classifications, including ICD-9, where this coding schedule is controlled by the NHS Centre for Coding and Classification. Read Codes cover such topics as occupations, signs and symptoms, investigations, diagnoses, treatments and therapies, drugs and appliances. Each clinical term in a clinical document is replaced by a Read Code when it is stored; when the clinical document is retrieved, the clinician is not presented with the code but with the clinical term.

receptor: A protein on the surface of a cell or the interior of a cell that binds with specific molecules. The binding may or may not affect the internal chemistry of the cell.

red flag: A change in a medical condition that could be a warning of a critical point in the life cycle of the medical condition. A clinician could identify a red flag during the patient's visit, or the patient could be told to look for a red flag and seek help upon the red flag occurring.

re-engineering: Rethinking and redesigning business processes to achieve quantum improvements in the performance of the business, which may be improvements in cost, quality, service or speed.

referral: Sending or directing a patient for consultation or treatment with another clinician or another medical department, usually where the referred-to clinician is a particular specialist physician and the referring clinician is a primary care physician. A referral involves a delegation of responsibility which should be followed up to ensure satisfactory care.

regenerative medicine: Development of artificial organs grown from tissues and cells (which often are stem cells).

ribosome: A structure within the cytoplasm of cells where the manufacture of protein could occur.

RNA (ribonucleic acid): "The genetic material of certain viruses (RNA viruses) and, in cellular organisms, the molecule that directs the middle steps of polypeptide, and later protein, production." (Microsoft ® Encarta ® 2007)

RNAi (RNA interference): A naturally occurring microRNA that can be used to knock down a protein. See "knock down."

scanned medical record form: A scanned paper medical record form that is given digitized index data to allow the scanned form to be displayed within an EPR (or a UPR) system.

secure health care network: A secure network that can directly interface UPRs with EPR systems.

significant health problem: A current, permanent or long-lasting disease or medical condition. Significant health problems appear in "clinical summaries."

somatic cell: All the cells in the human body excluding reproductive cells (e.g., eggs, sperm).

SNF (skilled nursing facility): A facility which provides inpatient skilled nursing care but does not require the level of care provided in a hospital.

specialist: A physician who works in a department not providing primary care, also known as a "specialty care physician."

specialty care: A classification of specialized fields of medical services, such as dermatology, urology, orthopedics, etc.

standard-of-care: Treatment that experts agree is appropriate, accepted and widely used.

stem cell: A cell that can incur unlimited division and which has the potential to differentiate into other types of cells.

synapse: A gap between the ends of two dendrites connected to different neurons.

synthetic biology: The application of genetic engineering to generate new biologic entities such as enzymes or vaccines or to redesign existing biological systems.

systems biology: Study of biological systems at the cellular level.

target cell: A cell that has a receptor that binds with a particular drug or hormone is called a "target cell" for that drug or hormone.

team-based care: "A highly disciplined [collection] of people brought together to perform tasks and functions that are too complex and critical for them to do alone or carry out independently of one another without serious consequences." (Lawrence 2003)

telemedicine: The use of interactive audio and visual links to enable remote healthcare practitioners to consult in "real time" with healthcare practitioners in distant medical centers.

tissue: "A group of associated, similarly structured cells that perform specialized functions for the survival of the organism." (Microsoft ® Encarta ® 2007)

TIFF (Tagged Image File Format): "a file format for storing images, including photographs and line art." (Wikipedia 2009)

(gene) transcription: A process that occurs in gene expression whereby the double stranded DNA opens up and the

DNA sequence in a gene is used as a template to produce a messenger RNA.

(gene) translation: A process that may occur in gene expression after gene transcription where the messenger RNA migrates to a ribosome in the cell's cytoplasm where information is used to create a polypeptide.

transfer: Change in medical care unit, hospital, medical staff, or responsible physician of an inpatient after hospitalization.

triage: Assessment of patients' medical problems to determine urgency and priority of care in the emergency department to determine which patient is to be seen next. Also the assessment of the medical problems of a single patient to determine the order of treatment of the medical problems.

TURP (Transurethral resection of the prostate): A procedure to treat benign prostatic hyperplasia where an instrument is inserted up the urethra to remove a section of the prostate blocking urine flow.

universal patient medical record (UPR): "A distributed patient medical record that summarizes and electronically combines all of a patient's medical information and would be available to all clinicians caring for the patient no matter where the clinician or patient is located in the world." (McGuire 2004)

universal patient health number: A term used by the ASTM for a patient identifier that is unique to an individual. (ASTM 2009)

virtual team: A group of health care workers that rely primarily or exclusively on electronic forms of communication to work together in the care of a patient. Members of a virtual team may not normally work together and may not even know each other.

wellness: The idea that healthy behaviors can increase longevity and protect against disease.

wrapper: Enclosing data by other data at the front and end to enable the enclosed data to be transported over a network. For example a PDF wrapper would be enclosed around DICOM data to enable the data to be sent over a network to another computer as if the whole of the data was PDF, but the program in the receiving computer would strip off the PDF wrapper and use the DICOM data.

XML (Extensible Markup Language): A text format for creating structured computer documents.

XSL (Extensible Stylesheet Language): A language used to describe how an XML document should be rendered (printed, displayed or heard).

CPSIA information can be obtained
at www.ICGtesting.com
Printed in the USA
LVOW04s0901190816

·500722LV00021B/260/P